1001
PEDIATRIC
TREATMENT
ACTIVITIES

Creative Ideas for
Therapy Sessions

1001
PEDIATRIC
TREATMENT
ACTIVITIES

Creative Ideas for
Therapy Sessions

Ayelet Danto, MS, OTR/L • Michelle Pruzansky, MS, OTR/L

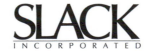

Published by: SLACK Incorporated
                  6900 Grove Road
                  Thorofare, NJ 08086 USA
                  Telephone: 856-848-1000
                  Fax: 856-848-6091
                  www.slackbooks.com

Contact SLACK Incorporated for more information about other books in this field or about the availability of our books from distributors outside the United States.

Financial Disclosure: Ayelet Danto and Michelle Pruzansky have no financial or proprietary interest in the materials presented herein.

Library of Congress Cataloging-in-Publication Data

Danto, Ayelet.
 1001 pediatric treatment activities : creative ideas for therapy sessions / Ayelet Danto, Michelle Pruzansky.
     p. ; cm.
 One thousand and one pediatric activities
 One thousand one pediatric activities
 Includes bibliographical references and index.
 ISBN 978-1-55642-968-2
 1. Psychomotor disorders in children--Exercise therapy. 2. Occupational therapy for children. I. Pruzansky, Michelle. II. Title.
III. Title: One thousand and one pediatric activities. IV. Title: One thousand one pediatric activities.
 [DNLM: 1. Occupational Therapy--methods--Handbooks. 2. Child--Handbooks. 3. Psychomotor Disorders--rehabilitation--Handbooks. 4. Psychomotor Disorders--therapy--Handbooks. WB 39]
 RJ506.P68D36 2011
 618.92'89165--dc22
                          2010043449

For permission to reprint material in another publication, contact SLACK Incorporated. Authorization to photocopy items for internal, personal, or academic use is granted by SLACK Incorporated provided that the appropriate fee is paid directly to Copyright Clearance Center. Prior to photocopying items, please contact the Copyright Clearance Center at 222 Rosewood Drive, Danvers, MA 01923 USA; phone: 978-750-8400; website: www.copyright.com; email: info@copyright.com
Printed in the United States of America.

Last digit is print number: 10 9 8 7 6 5 4 3

Dedications

For Jason, Samantha, and Ally, with love
-Michelle

In loving memory of my father, Azriel Golowa A"H, who took great pride in his
children's accomplishments.
-Ayelet

Contents

About the Authors

Ayelet Danto, MS, OTR/L, is an occupational therapist who has worked in various school settings with a broad range of diagnoses. She currently works in the Passaic public school system, primarily with children with pervasive developmental disorders and with autistic spectrum disorders. She received her bachelor's degree in psychology from Yeshiva University Stern College for Women and a master's degree in occupational therapy from Columbia University. She currently resides in Passaic, NJ, with her husband and children.

Michelle Pruzansky, MS, OTR/L, is a pediatric occupational therapist specializing in the treatment of children with autistic spectrum disorders. Michelle received her bachelor's degree from Yeshiva University Stern College for Women and her master's degree in occupational therapy from Columbia University. Michelle currently lives in Bergenfield, NJ, with her husband and children. She is the head therapist and clinical coordinator at school #19 in Passaic, NJ, and also works at the Department of Children and Families, Passaic Regional School.

Acknowledgments

We wanted to jointly thank all the children who modeled for us and patiently allowed us to photograph them time after time: Avraham Simcha, Moshe, Sarah, Aharon, Ronit, Samantha, Ally, Netanel, Yosi, Jillian, Josh, Shuey, Yonatan, Talia, Sarina, Tara, Aryeh, Brian W., Nadav, Brian L., Joel, and Justin. We are grateful for our coworkers, teachers, and friends at School #6 & School #19 in Passaic, NJ. We are especially thankful to Dinah Leiter for allowing us to use her equipment and private practice space at Kid Clan in Passaic, NJ. Dinah has not only served as an employer, but also as a friend. We would like to thank Debra Tupe, pediatric professor at Columbia University for taking the time to review our manuscript and provide us with insightful feedback that has helped strengthen our book. We also wanted to thank Neil B. Friedman, Esq., for his advice and continued legal services along the way. Last, we wanted to jointly thank Brien Cummings, our acquisitions editor at SLACK Incorporated, for helping make this book become a reality and for the countless hours of work he has spent on it.

We also wanted to give our individual thanks:

There have been many people that have greatly influenced me along my career path and throughout life. I wanted to personally thank each of them. My mother and father, Brenda and Bill Wiener, have always pushed me to be my best and never accepted anything less. It is because of them I have learned that through hard work and perseverance, no goal of mine is out of reach.

My wonderful mother- and father-in-law, Amy and Larry Pruzansky, have always been there to provide advice and support whenever needed, and for this I am truly grateful.

My extraordinary siblings deserve special mention for the many ways they have enriched my life. Tamar & Rony, Brian, Yisroel & Chani, Tara & Aryeh, and Talia.

I would also like to thank my co-author Ayelet, who helped make this book a reality with your hard work and dedication.

To my dear children, Samantha and Ally, you are a wonderful blessing. Raising you has been exciting, rewarding, and nothing short of joyous. You have taught me many important lessons and showed me the true meaning of unconditional love.

To my life partner and best friend—my husband, Jason. I know I can count on you to listen and guide me along life's journeys. I look up to you for your knowledge and valuable advice you always give me. I am truly blessed to have you in my life.

- *Michelle*

I would like to express my unending gratitude to God for giving us the abilities and opportunity to create this book.

I would like to thank my parents, Azriel A"H and Judith Golowa, for always encouraging and guiding me throughout my life and being so supportive of my career and the creation of this book.

I am grateful to my in-laws, Dr. Joseph and Marilyn Danto, for always expressing interest in the development of this publication and for always giving of their time and efforts to help whenever needed.

I would like to thank my siblings (and siblings-in-law), Dvora, Yosef, and Ahron & Rachel, Melissa & Moshe, Jeni & Akiva, and Ephy & Bracha for always showing interest and excitement for our book.

I would like to thank Michelle, my co-author. Her ambition and determination was a driving force to the completion of this book.

My children Avraham Simcha, Moshe, Sara, Aharon, and Nechama have always expressed excitement about "Mommy's book" and posed for countless pictures and retakes of pictures "just to help mommy." I know they are proud of their mother but that pales in comparison to how proud I am of them.

I would like to thank my husband, Netanel, for his unending love, support, encouragement, and proofreading, input and great advice in every aspect of this book. He is an inspiration to me in all aspects of my life.

- *Ayelet*

Introduction

As many pediatric therapists know, when working with children for extended periods of time in the same environment, it is quite challenging to find and develop new and exciting treatment activities. In order to be effective, therapists must not only treat specific impairments, but do so in a creative and resourceful manner that engages children and maintains their attention and interest. It is for this reason we developed this guidebook.

History

While working in a public school setting in a multi-disciplinary team of therapists, we found ourselves using the same activities over and over again. It became challenging for the therapists to constantly be coming up with fresh ideas. To make matters worse, many children noticed that they were engaging in the same activities session after session. Hearing "didn't we already play this game" or "this again?" was not encouraging. In an effort to find new ideas, we searched for different resources and books that could help with this problem. While we were able to find some resources that addressed a specific treatment area, we were not able to find any that comprehensively covered the gamut of treatment areas that were typically addressed in a pediatric setting. So, we decided to take action and do something about this problem.

We started by putting together a list of treatment areas that are typically addressed in pediatric therapy. We then began to compile lists of different and exciting activities for each treatment area with the help of other therapists from a variety of disciplines. Every day we would add new activities to our list. This "small list" began to evolve into a binder full of activities. Soon enough we began to realize that even the most creative and experienced therapist can really benefit from new ideas. That is when we decided to put our efforts toward publishing this book.

Purpose

The purpose of this book is to enhance resources available to therapists. This book serves to add to our profession's working knowledge and access to treatment activity ideas in a wide range of areas. This book is meant to be a quick and simple reference or handbook for any pediatric therapist looking for new ideas for a therapy session.

How to Use This Book

This book is intended to be used as a quick reference and not meant to provide a detailed activity analysis for the different topics addressed. The book was organized and written in a way that enables its user to quickly open it and skim a chapter for new ideas. The activities were carefully organized and written in simple language and with the intent of being as concise as possible.

While most activities can be explained in a short sentence, some activities require further explanation. Therefore, many activities in this book also are accompanied by a photograph to help further explain the intent and setup of the activity.

Contents and Organization

The information in this book is divided into seven sections, each with multiple chapters. Each chapter within a given section provides the following information:

- ✧ An introduction
- ✧ A brief description explaining the treatment topic
- ✧ An explanation of why a particular skill is important
- ✧ A list of compensatory strategies that may be employed by the child who is deficient in the particular skill

+ A list of treatment ideas and activities in which to engage, in order to work on the specific treatment goal
+ Examples of commercial products that can be used to address the treatment goal

Generally, treatment activities were placed in the most suitable sections; however, many activities addressed more than one goal at a time. For this reason, there were several activities that were listed in multiple sections.

Frame of Reference

Multiple frames of reference were used when compiling this book including the Biomechanical Frame of Reference and the Sensory Motor Model (Giroux Bruce & Borg, 2002). The intent of this organization was to offer a wide variety of easy-to-access activities to choose from in many different areas. However, the purpose of this book is not intended to dictate the way treatment is given, but rather provide therapists with the tools necessary to come up with different treatment activities. It is up to the treating therapist to determine the appropriate frame of reference to use with each individual child.

Who Should Use This Book

This book was written with the intent to be used primarily by pediatric occupational and physical therapists. However, this book may also be useful for a teacher, psychologist, or other pediatric educators.

Many activities provided in this book require skilled and experienced knowledge of working with children and may be harmful or ineffective if used in the wrong way. It is therefore important that any laymen using this book consult with a physical or occupational therapist before performing any of the suggested activities. It is also important that if any activity is unclear, it is should be reviewed with a trained pediatric occupational or physical therapist.

Populations Intended For

This book was written with the intent to be used among a wide range of populations and pediatric settings. Specifically, these settings include a pediatric clinic, school-based setting, hospital, and home-based therapy. When writing this book, a wide variety of diagnoses and conditions were kept in mind including, but not limited to, children with fine motor and gross motor delays, traumatic injuries, congenital abnormalities, perinatal injuries, Attention-deficit hyperactivity disorder, Attention-deficit disorder, cerebral palsy, autistic spectrum disorders, dyspraxia, global delays, learning disabilities, Down syndrome and other chromosomal disorders.

About Play

As mentioned earlier, particularly when working with children with disabilities, each child displays different strengths and weaknesses and does not necessarily develop according to a defined schedule. However it is helpful to remember the different stages of play that children normally engage in at different points of development as a reference point. This can be of assistance in choosing age/developmentally appropriate play activities for a child from the variety of play activities included in this book.

Nancy Takata developed play epochs under the leadership of Mary Reilly, the famous occupational therapist who was instrumental in developing the occupational behavior frame of reference (Parham & Fazio, 1997).

Takata's play epochs can be understood in the explanation below (ages identified are approximate) (1974):

+ *Sensorimotor age 0-2:* Solitary play (no peer interaction) involving motor and sensation such as peek-a-boo, patty cake, imitation of caregivers, container play, exploring objects, practicing new motor skills and simple problem solving.
+ *Symbolic and simple constructive age 2-4:* Beginning of make believe and pretend play, shift from solitary play to parallel play (playing side by side with peer with little or no interaction). Building simple constructions that represent another object or situation. Practicing climbing and running.

- *Dramatic, complex constructive, and pregame age 4-7:* More social participation. Associative play (participating in group with a shared activity), dramatic role playing enacting daily experiences, social roles, fairy tales, and myths. Skill in activities requiring hand dexterity. Daredevil activities involving strength and skill outdoors. Constructions are realistic and complex. Verbal humor, creates rhymes.
- *Game age 7-12:* Games with rules. Fascination with rules. Masters established rules and makes up new ones. Risk taking in games. Concern with peer status. Friendship groups important. Interest in sports and formal groups. Cooperative play (cooperates with peers in highly organized activity). Interest in how things work, nature, crafts.
- *Recreational age 12-16:* Formal peer group orientation, teamwork, cooperation, respect for rules, games that challenge skills, competitive sports, service clubs. Realistic constructive projects and complex manual skills.

Although this information is helpful, when choosing a play activity for a child it is of utmost importance to keep in mind the preferences and desires of the particular child with whom you are working.

Final Things to Consider

- *Grading:* Grading an activity is the ability to modify an activity's challenge level in order to appropriately suit the skill level of a child. While some methods of gradation are provided within this book, for the most part it is left up to the treating therapist to properly grade the activity to an appropriate level of challenge. Grading an activity must be done on an individual basis, keeping the different components of the activity in mind, along with the different strengths and weaknesses of the child.
- *Repetition:* Repetitive practice of a skill helps a child improve in an area and generalize the skill to other areas. It is for this reason that multiple activities and ideas are provided for each treatment topic addressed.
- *Fatigue:* When supervising children engaged in different treatment activities it is important to watch the child's level of fatigue. Pushing a child too hard can be unsafe and ineffective from a therapeutic standpoint. This is especially true for many children with low muscle tone and other medical diagnoses.

Conclusion

It has been both rewarding and hard work putting together this book over the past four years. It is our hope that our fellow clinicians benefit from the activities presented and make therapy more fun for the children with whom they work. We urge readers to use caution and sound clinical reasoning when implementing the activities provided. We challenge clinicians to continuously employ innovative strategies and expand upon what we have presented in this book. We wish all therapists the best of luck in their future endeavors!

Important Warning and Disclaimer

The authors of this book are not responsible for use or misuse of the treatment activities provided. All activities provided should be closely supervised by a trained occupational or physical therapist or under the guidance of one. Before implementing any activities provided in this book, one must first check for any medical contraindications. Additionally, several activities involve the use of food. It is important to check for any food allergies before using food in an activity.

It also is important to be aware of toys or objects that may pose a choking hazard to infants and small children. The general rule is that the size of the toy should not fit through a toilet paper roll, but it is best to always consult a pediatrician.

Additionally, before beginning treatment with any child, it is always important to become familiar with the child's background information specifically related to any medical conditions or diagnoses that may have accompanying contraindications or sequelae that may adversely affect a child in a specific activity or exercise.

Finally, there are many activities throughout this book that involve the use of therapeutic handling techniques. It is important that the therapist be skilled in proper handling techniques in order to safely and effectively implement the chosen activity. In order to become familiar with these handling techniques, the therapist should contact a trained pediatric occupational or physical therapist familiar with the specific population of interest.

SENSORY INTEGRATION

Sensory integration is the ability of the brain and body to take in information through the senses and interpret it into meaningful information (Ayres, 2005). The different senses include vision, touch, taste, smell, hearing, the vestibular sense (sense of movement), and the proprioceptive sense (sense of where the body is in space). When the brain does not properly interpret information brought in by the senses, the result will be a sensory integration dysfunction (SID). The following section will include activities geared toward addressing SID.

A child with SID may either seek out or avoid different sensory experiences, including movement, sights, touch, and sounds. Another manifestation of SID is when sensory information is not being properly interpreted by the brain and body, causing a child to be clumsy and have difficulty learning new motor tasks (Ayres, 2005). Additionally, a child may exhibit what appears as negative behaviors in an attempt to organize incoming sensory information.

For example, imagine Billy, a little 6-year-old boy who acts overly rough with his friends and exhibits hyperactive behaviors in school. Billy always seems to be getting in trouble, cannot keep up in Phys-Ed, and always seems to be one step behind in the classroom. Billy's teachers are annoyed with him, his classmates will not play with him, and his parents are frustrated.

In contrast to Billy, another child with SID may withdraw from peers or refuse to participate in classroom activities. When a child has difficulty processing sensory information, daily functioning in many areas are affected. However, children generally react differently to SID and the same areas are not always affected.

While there are many components to sensory integration, this section will focus on some of the main areas affected in children. These specifically include proprioception, motor planning, pressure modulation, bilateral integration/crossing midline, vestibular processing, tactile sensitivity, and oral motor difficulties. These topics will be addressed further in the upcoming chapters.

PROPRIOCEPTIVE ACTIVITIES

Proprioception is a sense that tells a person the location and orientation of one's body and limbs during stationary and movement activities (Ayres, 2005, p. 41). Body awareness is the awareness of where one's body is in space in relation to the environment and to one's self. Body awareness is greatly affected by proprioception. It is necessary to have a strong proprioceptive sense in order to easily perform motor activities in a coordinated fashion and navigate smoothly through one's environment. Many children that appear clumsy and uncoordinated have decreased body awareness and are often unsuccessful in executing an unfamiliar motor task.

Heavy work, deep pressure, and resistive activities provide input to the receptors within our muscles, which give our bodies information as to where they are in space (Ayres, 2005, p. 144). This chapter provides numerous heavy work, deep pressure, and resistive activities that strengthen the proprioceptive sense. Proprioceptive input can also help calm a child and help the child focus and attend to a desired activity.

When choosing a proprioceptive activity, it is important to first identify the needs of the child. While one overly active child may respond well to deep pressure, another child may find this sort of input confining and would respond better to a heavy work activity.

Danto, A., & Pruzansky, M. *1001 Pediatric Treatment Activities:
Creative Ideas for Therapy Sessions* (pp. 3-18).
© 2011 SLACK Incorporated

Proprioceptive Activities

Cleanup/Set-Up Activities

+ Child removes chairs from table and places them on top of table during cleanup.
+ Child drags and rearranges small tables, desks, chairs, and other small furniture in the room.
+ Child hangs up large mats or pulls them toward one side of the room.

Deep Pressure Activities

+ Bear hugs: Therapist gives child a large hug, wrapping arms all the way around child, maintaining constant and firm pressure.
+ Mummy wrap game: Therapist wraps child tightly in a sheet, blanket, or a towel. Therapist tucks the end of the material in and has child walk across the room without letting the sheet/blanket/towel fall to the ground.
+ Therapist ties two children together with Lycra material and then has them walk across the room.
+ Therapist massages child's back and feet.
+ Vibrations: Child uses an Innergizer or another vibrating machine (Figure 1-1). (Refer to user's manual for safety precautions and contraindications.)

FIGURE 1-1

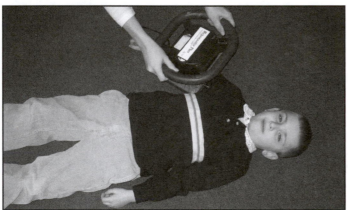

+ Brushing protocol: Refer to Wilbarger's brushing protocol[1] for instructions (Wilbarger & Wilbarger, 1991).
  ◇ Therapist brushes child according to brushing protocol.
  ◇ Older children can be taught to brush themselves (Figure 1-2).

FIGURE 1-2

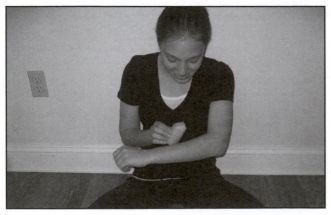

[1] Patricia Wilbarger, M.Ed., OTR, FAOTA, an internationally recognized occupational therapist and clinical psychologist who is a leading expert in the area of sensory defensiveness, developed this technique. Please refer to this reference on the Reference page for a detailed description on how to perform this treatment protocol.

◆ Joint compressions: Refer to Wilbarger's brushing protocol for instructions (Wilbarger & Wilbarger, 1991).

◆ Lycra swing: The material in a Lycra swing surrounds the child's body and provides deep pressure. Different Lycra swing activities include:

   ✧ Therapist swings child in Lycra swing (Figure 1-3).

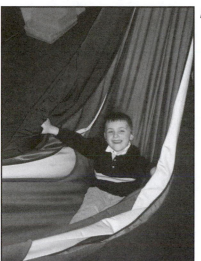

FIGURE 1-3

   ✧ Therapist plays peek-a-boo with child hidden in swing.

   ✧ Child climbs up the swing and slides down—only with long Lycra swing (Figure 1-4).

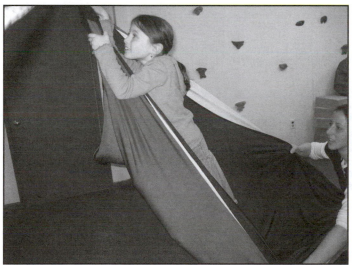

FIGURE 1-4

✦ Body sock: Therapist places child in a body sock and has child (Figure 1-5):

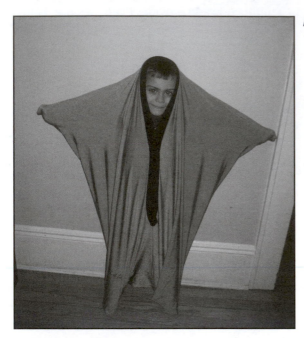

FIGURE 1-5

   ✧ Walk around the room.
   ✧ Play "Simon Says."
   ✧ Play "Patty-Cake."
✦ Quadruped activities: Child goes into quadruped position and:
   ✧ Colors on a large oak tag (Figure 1-6).

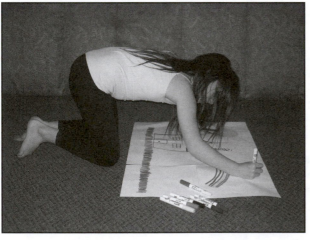

FIGURE 1-6

   ✧ Places pegs into a peg board on the floor or on a slightly raised surface.
   ✧ Assembles a puzzle.
   ✧ Maintains quadruped in a stationary position and counts to ten.
✦ "Hot Dog" and "Sandwich" games: Therapist "smushes" child with big pillows and has child pretend to be a hot dog while the pillows are the buns. Therapist should use careful judgment when "squishing" child and providing deep pressure.
✦ Ball pit games:
   ✧ Child crashes into the ball pit.
   ✧ Child hides self underneath the balls and then the therapist tries to find the child.

✦ Crab walking: Child crab walks across the room (Figure 1-7).

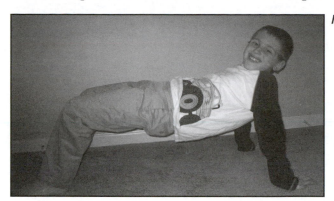

FIGURE 1-7

✦ Wheelbarrow walking: Child wheelbarrow walks across the room (Figure 1-8).

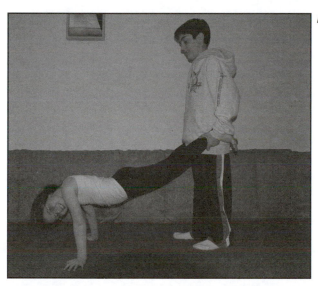

FIGURE 1-8

✦ Child wheelbarrow walks up ramp and then the therapist pulls the child down the ramp by the legs.
✦ Push-ups: Child performs different push-ups including:
  ◇ Regular floor push-ups (Figure 1-9).

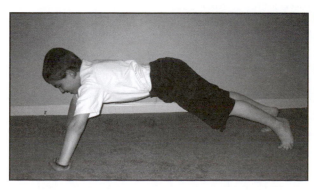

FIGURE 1-9

✧ Half push-ups with knees touching floor (Figure 1-10).

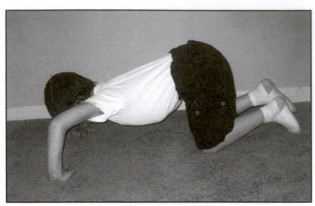

FIGURE 1-10

✧ Wall push-ups (Figure 1-11).

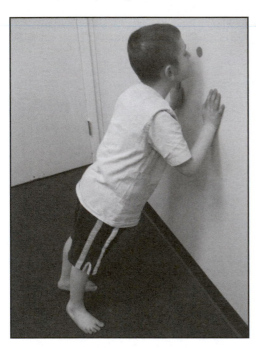

FIGURE 1-11

✧ Couch push-ups: Child lies on a couch on belly, hanging over the edge. Child places arms on the floor and pushes off the floor keeping lower body on the couch (Figure 1-12).

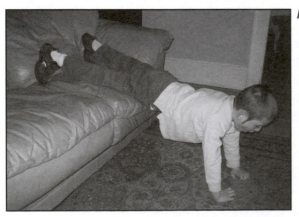

FIGURE 1-12

❖ Chair push-ups: Child sits on a chair, grabs each side of the chair with hands, locks elbows, pushes down, all while keeping bottom seated on chair (Figure 1-13).

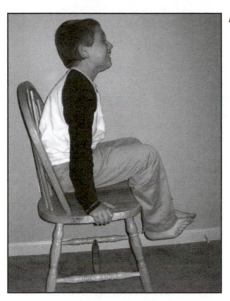

Figure 1-13

✦ Chin-ups: Child pulls self up on chin-up bar (Figure 1-14).

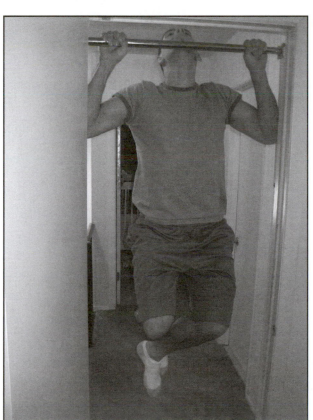

Figure 1-14

✦ Controlled pillow fights: Child and therapist take turns "pushing" each other with large pillows. Specific rules and guidelines of this game should be made clear in advance and the game should be terminated if the child becomes too rowdy or is not following the rules (Figure 1-15).

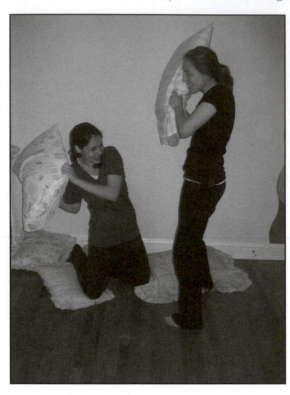

FIGURE 1-15

Activities Utilizing Weighted Equipment

Please note: Although as of yet there are no standardized guidelines, many recommend that therapists should use approximately 5% of the child's total body weight when placing weights in weighted garments (VandenBerg, 2001; Reichow, Barton, Neely Sewell, Good, Wolery, 2010).

✦ Therapist places weights in child's shirt and pant pockets.
✦ Child wears ankle and wrist weights during an activity.
✦ Therapist places a weighted lap pad on child during a seated activity.
✦ Child wears a weighted vest.
✦ Child lies in prone position (on belly) and therapist places a weighted blanket over child's back.
✦ Child plays catch with a weighted ball.

Heavy Work Activities

✦ Therapist places heavy objects on a scooter or in a wheelbarrow and the child pushes it around the room.
✦ Therapist places several text books in child's backpack and the child carries the heavy objects across the room.
✦ Therapist and child take turns giving "rides." Therapist sits on a chair with wheels and child gives a "ride." Therapist and child then switch positions and therapist pulls child around the room.

✦ Parachute games: Child sits in the center of a parachute while another child pulls the parachute around with an adult assisting (Figure 1-16).

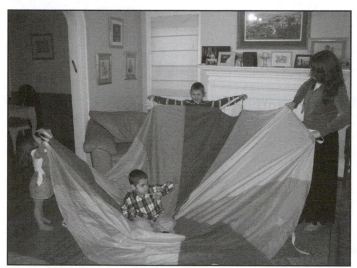

FIGURE 1-16

✦ Child lies on belly on a scooter board and propels himself around the room.

✦ Child lies on belly on a scooter board and pulls himself up a ramp.

✦ Child lies on belly on a scooter board and holds onto a bungee cord or jump rope and gets pulled by therapist. (An alternative method of this game would be to have child prone on the scooter board, tie a jump rope around a door knob, and have the child pull himself back and forth.)

✦ Child sits on swing and holds onto one end of a hula hoop. Therapist holds onto the other end and pulls child back and forth on the swing (Figure 1-17).

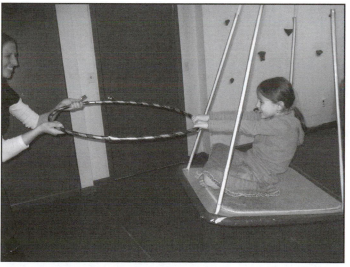

FIGURE 1-17

✦ Squeeze a squeeze toy: Child squeezes a stress ball, Koosh ball, or other sensory ball.

✦ Velcro toys: Child pulls apart different toys fastened together by heavy-duty Velcro.

✦ Child pretends to be as strong as a superhero with special powers. Child then pushes against the walls and pretends that the walls are moving.

✦ Leaning Tower of Pisa game: Two children (or therapist and child) face each other and place hands palm-to-palm. Therapist and child lean into each other and hold this position for as long as possible, pretending to be the Leaning Tower of Pisa (Figure 1-18).

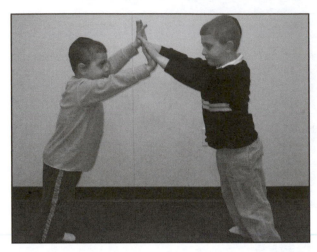

FIGURE 1-18

✦ Modified wrestling: Therapist faces child. Therapist and child interlock hands and lean in toward each other. The object of this game is to see who can keep their balance longer without falling backward or to the side. This game should be closely supervised to make sure nobody gets hurt and should only be played with a child that will not become overly rowdy.

✦ "Row, Row, Row Your Boat" game: In this game, child sits on the floor, facing either the therapist or another child, each holding onto one end of a jump rope (position I) or onto each other's wrists (position II). As both sing the song, one person leans back as the other leans forward and then the opposite.

  ◇ Position I (Figure 1-19).

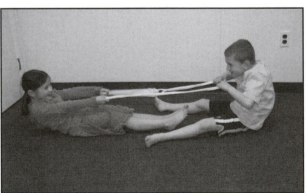

FIGURE 1-19

  ◇ Position II (Figure 1-20).

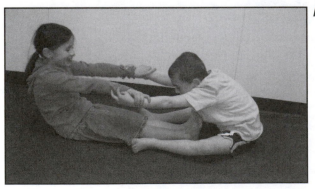

FIGURE 1-20

✦ Therapy ball activities:

   ✧ Therapist rolls a very large therapy ball toward the child quickly. Child must stop it with hands and then push it back toward the therapist very hard and quickly.

   ✧ Child pushes against a large therapy ball while another child or therapist gives resistance from the other side (Figure 1-21).

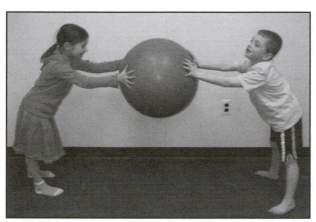

Figure 1-21

   ✧ Child pushes a large therapy ball through a Lycra tunnel. Make sure that the therapy ball is larger than the walls of the tunnel so that the child will have to use resistance to push the ball through (Figures 1-22 and 1-23).

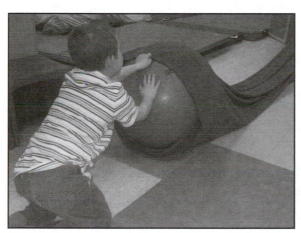

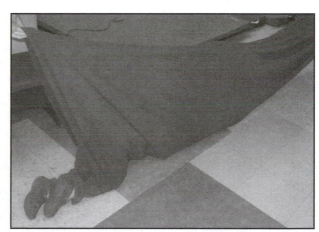

Figure 1-22   *Figure 1-23*

   ✧ Child holds a medium-sized therapy ball in the air with arms and legs while lying on back. Therapist tries to take the ball away and has child hold onto the ball as hard as possible.

✦ Door opener: Child opens a large, heavy door and then keeps it open while others walk through.

✦ Bubble wrap:

   ✧ Child pops bubbles on bubble wrap paper.

   ✧ Child jumps up and down on a sheet of large bubble wrap paper.

✦ Stapling: Child staples papers onto a bulletin board with adult supervision or assists in stapling stacks of papers that need to be stapled together.

✦ Theraputty exercises:

   ✧ Child pinches, pulls, and squeezes Theraputty.

   ✧ Child hides different objects in the putty and then tries to find them as quickly as possible. (This activity can be made more exciting by using a timer to see how quickly the child can work and then see if the child can break his own record or by letting the child keep a prize found in the putty.)

✦ Theraband exercises:
   ❖ Child places Theraband under both feet and pulls up with both arms at each side (Figure 1-24).

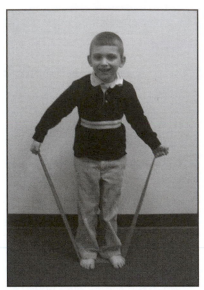

FIGURE 1-24

   ❖ Child holds Theraband with both hands at chest level and pulls Theraband apart to each side (Figure 1-25).

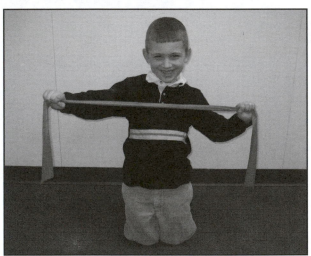

FIGURE 1-25

⬧ Child holds Theraband behind back and pulls out with both hands (Figure 1-26).

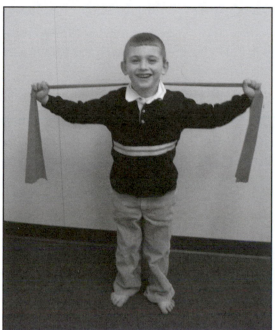

Figure 1-26

  ⬧ Therapist ties Theraband to the side of a chair. Child pulls and tugs at Theraband throughout therapy session or during class as needed.
  ⬧ Therapist ties Theraband around both front legs of a chair and lets child kick back at Theraband as needed in the therapy session or the classroom.
✦ Child colors on a chalkboard or dry-erase board and then washes and dries the board, pushing very hard onto the surface.
✦ Tug-of-war (Figure 1-27).

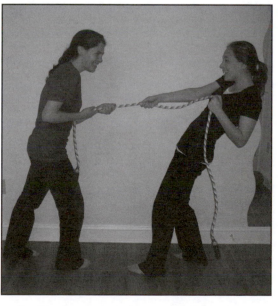

Figure 1-27

✦ Trapeze bar: Child hangs onto trapeze bar by holding on with his hands or hanging upside-down and hanging from his legs.

Climbing Activities

◆ Child climbs up a ladder in the therapy room.
◆ Child climbs up the wall with legs: Place child in a quadruped position with child's feet next to the wall. Have child walk feet slowly up the wall so that the body is in a 90 degree angle with the wall (Figure 1-28).

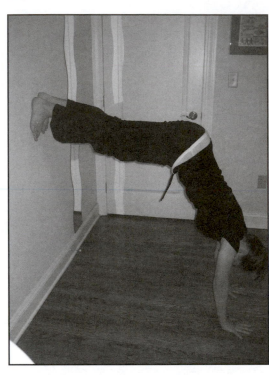

FIGURE 1-28

◆ Child swings across on monkey bars in the playground (Figure 1-29).

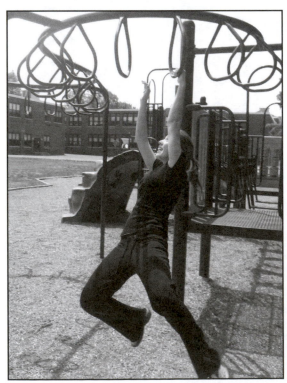

FIGURE 1-29

✦ Child hangs on single monkey bar in the playground (Figure 1-30).

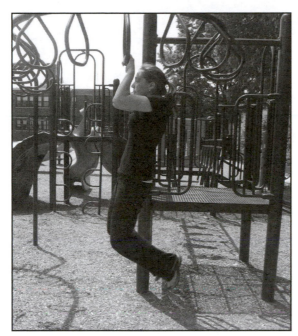

FIGURE 1-30

Jumping Activities

Should be done under close supervision of a therapist.

✦ "Pop Goes the Weasel": Child squats on the floor and sings "Pop Goes the Weasel." Every time the word "pop" is sung, child should jump up.

✦ "Five Little Monkeys": Child squats on the floor and sings "Five Little Monkeys Jumping on a Bed." The child should jump up and down during this part of the song. Child should then crash into a large pillow or bean bag at the point in the song: "one fell off and bumped his head."

✦ Relay races: Have child or group of children frog jump from one end of the room to the other.

✦ Child jumps on a trampoline and then crashes into big pillows.

✦ Child jumps up and down on either a mattress or large pillows/bean bags.

✦ Child jumps off of a high surface into a large bean bag pillow.

Baking Activities

✦ Knead dough: Therapist and child perform a baking activity that requires kneading dough (cookies, pizza, bread). Child uses hands to knead the dough.

✦ Therapist uses a recipe that requires mixing of heavy dough or another resistive substance and has child mix the batter with a baking utensil.

Special Foods to Eat

Be aware of any allergies or special diets before giving child any food.

Additionally, rule out any feeding or swallowing problems before using food in treatment.

✦ Therapist provides child with crunchy/hard foods, including oat bars, crunchy cereal, etc.

✦ Therapist provides child with chewy foods, including bagels, gum, licorice, chewy bars, peanut butter, etc.

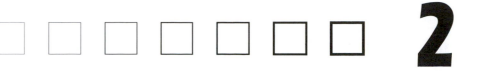

MOTOR PLANNING

Motor planning refers to the ability to plan and execute an unfamiliar or complicated motor task or novel motor experience in a coordinated fashion. A child with motor planning difficulties may appear clumsy and uncoordinated. Difficulty with motor planning is often associated with decreased body awareness (Ayres, 1965). Children with poor body awareness have a decreased sense of where their body parts/limbs are in relation to each other and their environment. Additionally, perceptual and cognitive skills may impact a child's motor planning and subsequent body awareness.

Activities that provide children with deep pressure or heavy work help increase body awareness by "waking up" the muscles and providing the muscles with a better sense of where they are in relation to the rest of the body. When performing challenging motor planning activities (such as those provided in this chapter), it is important to precede these activities with deep pressure and/or heavy work. Refer to Chapter 1 on proprioceptive activities for more ideas.

The activities provided in this chapter will challenge and help improve a child's motor planning skills. A child may take several attempts and require physical or verbal assistance in order to perform these activities successfully. As with any therapeutic activity, the more a child practices, the better the child will be able to generalize the gained skills into other new and challenging activities.

Danto, A., & Pruzansky, M. *1001 Pediatric Treatment Activities:*
Creative Ideas for Therapy Sessions (pp. 19-28).
© 2011 SLACK Incorporated

Motor Planning Treatment Activities

Ball Activities

✦ "Neck ball": Child holds a ball with neck and passes it along to another child's neck without using hands (Figure 2-1).

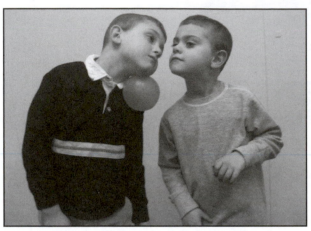

FIGURE 2-1

✦ Tic-Tock-Tire: Therapist hangs up a suspended tire swing (a hula hoop is ok too) and swings it from side to side. Place a bucket full of small items (bean bags, koosh balls, etc.) on the floor to the side of the child. Have child pick up one item at a time and throw it through the moving tire without letting it touch the tire.

   ✧ In order to make this activity more challenging have child stand on a balance board while throwing the bean bags.

   ✧ In order to downgrade this activity, keep the tire still or move it ever so slightly (Figure 2-2).

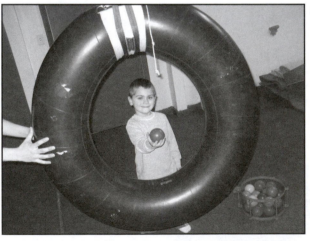

FIGURE 2-2

✦ This activity can also be played in the form of catch. Have child stand on one side of the tire and therapist on the other side. Play catch with a small ball while keeping the tire swaying from side to side.

Body Positioning

- ✦ Imitation of different body positions:
  - ✧ Child tries to imitate another child or therapist's position.
  - ✧ Child plays "Simon Says" imitating different positions.
  - ✧ Child is shown photographs of people in different positions and tries to place self in same position as person in the photograph.
- ✦ Imitation of different finger and hand positions: Therapist faces child and positions own hands or fingers in a specific position. Hold the position and have child try and create a mirror image of the position.
- ✦ "Animal walk": Therapist assigns child an animal and then has child assume the different animal positions. Child then walks across the room in these positions. Some examples include frog, kangaroo, snake, elephant, lion, bear, and rabbit (Figures 2-3 and 2-4).

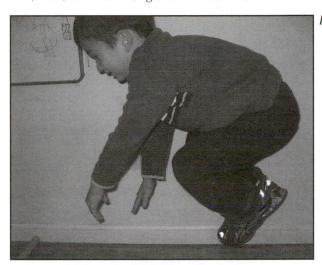

FIGURE 2-3

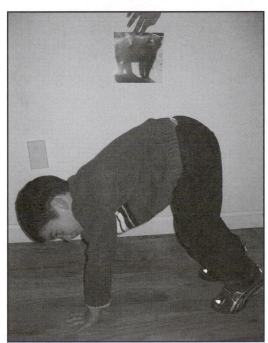

FIGURE 2-4

✦ "Statue game": This activity can be played one-to-one or in a group. Therapist designates a "leader" and has leader pretend to be different statues. Child must then try and imitate the different statues and positions.

✦ Body letter making: Therapist places children in groups of 2 to 4 people. Therapist has each group pick a letter (A to Z) out of a hat. Therapist tells children in a specific group to try and place their bodies into the correct positions to make the letter on the floor. (This game can also be played individually, but will only work with some of the alphabet letters).

Body Movement Games

✦ Child points to and labels different body parts upon request. This activity can be made more exciting if played to a song. Some examples of songs include "Head, shoulders, knees, and toes" "If You're Happy and You Know It (... touch your nose, head, etc.)." (Singing these songs in front of a mirror may help if child is having trouble touching the correct body part.)

✦ "Hokey Pokey": Therapist sings the Hokey Pokey song while helping child put the correct body part in and out of the circle. (This game can also be helpful for right/left orientation.)

✦ Hopscotch: Therapist creates a hopscotch board on the floor with masking tape (or sidewalk chalk outside). Child plays hopscotch and concentrates, when jumping, on opening, closing, and alternating feet onto correct spaces.

✦ Child climbs on top of a therapy ball and uses a trapeze bar to climb into a Lycra swing. In order to upgrade this activity, tell the child which foot/arm to put in first (Figure 2-5).

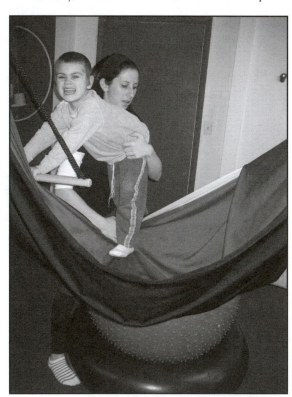

FIGURE 2-5

✦ Elbow to knee: Child raises left knee and taps it with right elbow, then repeats on opposite knee with other hand (Figures 2-6 and 2-7).

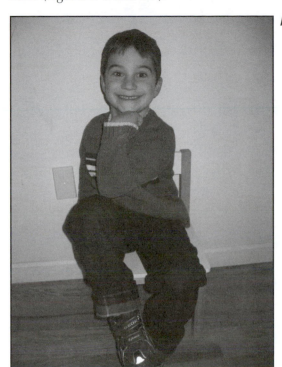

Figure 2-6

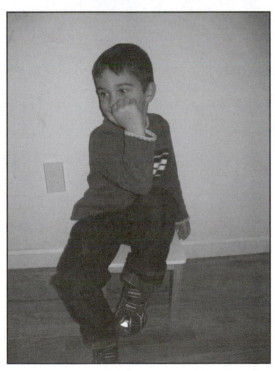

Figure 2-7

✦ Child sings "The Itsy Bitsy Spider" along with therapist. Child brings right index finger to the left thumb and left index finger to the right thumb, then flip fingers up in alternating fashion (Figures 2-8 and 2-9).

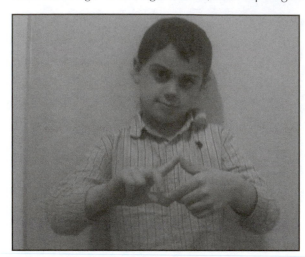

FIGURE 2-8

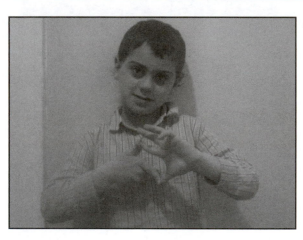

FIGURE 2-9

✦ Child self-pumps on frog swing or on playground swing.

✦ Therapist holds up a series of hula hoops and child crawls/walks through them without letting the hoops touch body. Child can also try and walk through the tire swing without touching it (Figure 2-10).

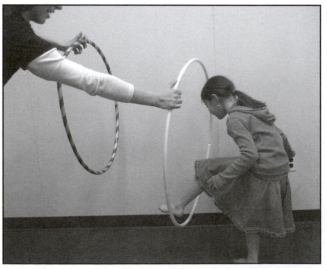

FIGURE 2-10

✦ Child spins a hula hoop around each wrist, starting and stopping every few seconds on cue (Figure 2-11).

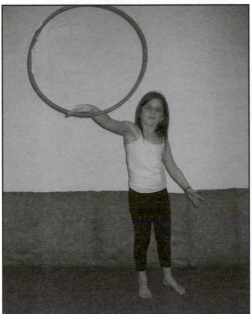

Figure 2-11

✦ Child performs multistep obstacle courses which can include:
  ✧ Climbing toys
  ✧ Slides
  ✧ Crash mats
  ✧ Bean bags
  ✧ Ball pits
  ✧ Balance beam/balance board
  ✧ Trampolines
  ✧ Suspended equipment

✦ Child climbs on unfamiliar playground equipment (Figures 2-12 through 2-15).

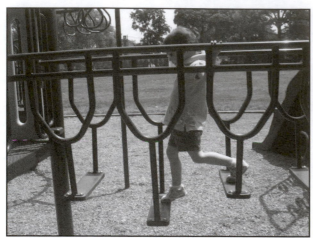

FIGURE 2-12

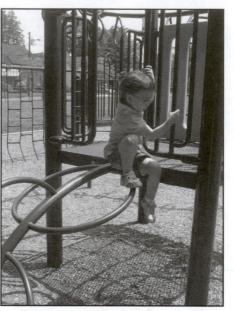

FIGURE 2-13

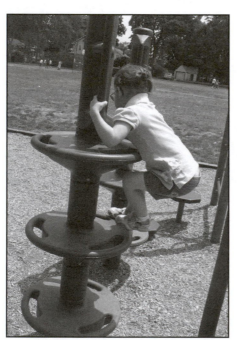

FIGURE 2-14

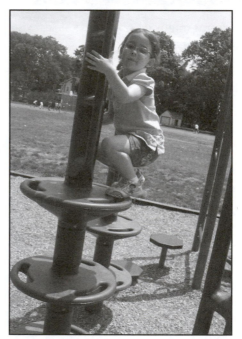

FIGURE 2-15

✦ Therapist places toy a small distance from the child (developmental age 7-12 months) (Cottrell, 2004, p. 19). While sitting on the floor, therapist then puts out his/her leg as an obstacle for the child to crawl over in order to get to the desired toy.

    ◇ The therapist can also place other obstacles such as pillows or soft wedges for the child to crawl over.

Activities With Eyes Closed

✦ Child closes eyes and therapist touches a specific body part on the child, applying consistent pressure for one to two seconds and then removes hand. Child then opens eyes and identifies the body part touched.

✦ Therapist places a red dot on the wall at eye level with the child. Child moves index finger from nose to the dot and back three consecutive times. Child then tries to perform this activity with eyes closed.

✦ Therapist draws a number/letter/shape with finger on child's back. Child tries to guess what was drawn.

   ✧ This activity can also be played on child's hands: Have child close eyes and then therapist draws a number/letter/shape on the back of the child's hand. Child then guesses what was drawn.

   ✧ This activity can be downgraded by giving child a choice of two possible guesses of things that were drawn.

✦ "Hide and Seek": Therapist and child play together. (This activity requires child to completely cover entire body, which helps increase body awareness to all the different parts of the body. This is because the child must pay attention to body parts that are occluded from vision.)

Rolling

✦ Child rolls on a mat and keeps body straight.

✦ Log roll game: Child rolls on mat. When therapist says stop, child must freeze and say if he/she is on back, belly, or side.

Running, Skipping, Jumping

✦ Child performs a running jump through tire swing. (Lower the swing so that the child is able to easily jump through.)

✦ Therapist teaches child how to skip and gallop.

✦ Child practices jumping rope (Figure 2-16).

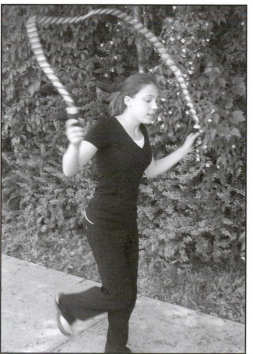

FIGURE 2-16

COMMERCIALLY AVAILABLE PRODUCTS

✦ "Twister"

✦ "Jenga"

✦ "Skip It"

✦ "WOGGLER"

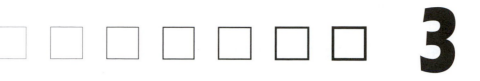

PRESSURE MODULATION

Pressure modulation is the ability of the body and joints to know how hard or lightly something should be touched. Poor pressure modulation can be manifested in many areas from self-care to play activities. For example, a child with decreased pressure modulation may be unable to push together or pull apart toys. The child may also not know the appropriate amount of pressure to use with writing utensils or how hard to squeeze glue bottles. This may cause the child to break pencil tips, squeeze too much toothpaste onto a toothbrush, or be unable to squeeze hard enough to get glue to come out of a glue bottle. There may even be social implications of poor pressure modulation, as a child may be unknowingly overly aggressive with his/her peers.

There are many activities and exercises that can help a child improve pressure modulation. The exercises provided in this chapter require a child to grade his/her force in order to be successful with that activity. Also of significance to note is that when performing an activity requiring the use of graded force, a therapist can upgrade the activity by placing a balance demand on the child in addition to the pressure modulation exercise itself. This is because a child requires more refined and precise pressure grading when placed on dynamic surfaces or during movement activities.

Danto, A., & Pruzansky, M. *1001 Pediatric Treatment Activities: Creative Ideas for Therapy Sessions* (pp. 29-34).
© 2011 SLACK Incorporated

Pressure Modulation Activities

Sports

+ There are several sports that can be played that require precise pressure modulation in order to be played successfully. Some of these sports include basketball, volleyball, miniature golf, ping pong, and billiards/pool.
+ Child throws a ball against the wall and catches it.
    ◇ Upgrade this activity by having child stand on a balance beam when throwing the ball.
+ Child throws a ball to a Velcro bull's-eye target (Figure 3-1).

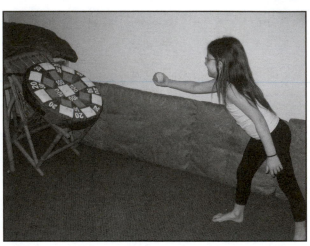

FIGURE 3-1

+ Balloon volleyball: Child hits balloon toward therapist with either a racquet or hands. Child tries to keep balloon from touching the floor for as long as possible.
+ Horseshoe toss: Therapist places stakes or sticks onto the floor or in the ground outside. Therapist provides child with horseshoes and has child toss the horseshoes onto the sticks.
+ Ring toss: Therapist places cones on floor and provides child with rings or hula hoops. Child then tosses rings onto cones.
+ Darts: Child shoots darts onto wall or a bull's-eye.
    ◇ The child can stand further or closer to the wall in order to upgrade or downgrade the activity respectively.
+ Skee-Ball: Child plays Skee-Ball if the equipment is available or therapist can simulate a Skee-Ball setup.

Craft Projects

+ Squeeze glue from a bottle onto a line.
    ◇ Sample Project—"Rainbow Making": Therapist gives each child a black and white rainbow. (See p. 212 of Appendix for sample template of project.) Child squeezes glue onto one line at a time and then sprinkles glitter on that line. Child proceeds to glue the following line and sprinkle it with a different color glitter.
+ Puff paint: Child creates craft projects using puff paint. Therapist reminds child that if too much pressure is applied to the tube, too much paint may come out.
+ Tin foil writing: Child writes name or makes a picture with toothpicks on a piece of tin foil and tries not to rip the tin foil.

- Shading projects:
  - Coin shading: Child places a quarter or another coin under a thin white piece of paper (not construction paper). Therapist provides child with a pencil and child lightly rubs pencil over the paper on top of the coin. A light imprint of the coin should show up on the paper.
  - Letter/shape shading: Therapist places cut out letters or other shapes from poster board and places them under the paper and has child shade the paper with a pencil or crayon.
  - Leaf shading: Therapist places leaves under a thin white piece of paper and has child lightly shade on top of the paper with a pencil or crayons.
- Picture making: Child draws the same picture three times with either a crayon or a pencil. One time the child should draw it as hard as possible, the second time should be as soft as possible, and the third time should be a middle amount of pressure. For smaller children who cannot understand this task, have them just draw three lines (hard, soft, medium).
- Cookie decorating: Child squeezes icing onto cookies in order to decorate them.

Recreational Children's Games

- Squeeze toys: Child squeezes a rocket launcher toy toward a target on the floor (Figures 3-2 through 3-4).

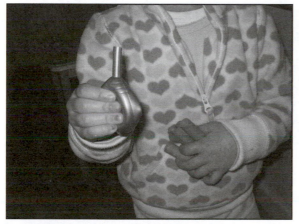

FIGURE 3-2

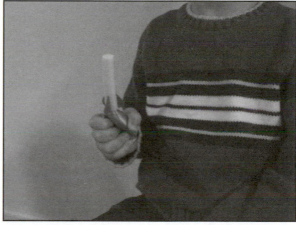

FIGURE 3-3

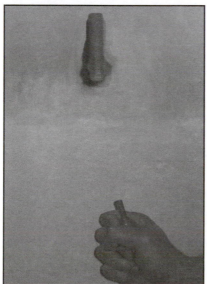

FIGURE 3-4

- Pop beads: Child pushes together and pulls apart pop beads.
- Child builds a tower with wooden blocks, trying not to allow the tower to fall.
- Dominos: Child creates a long line of dominos on a flat surface and then tips the last domino to watch the domino effect. It may be necessary to assist child in this task in order to make sure the child does not accidentally knock a domino over too early (Figures 3-5 through 3-7).

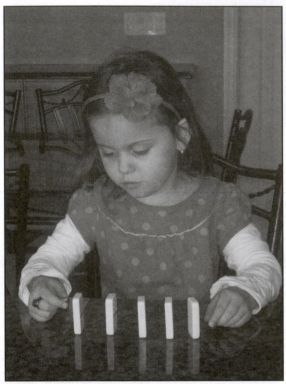

FIGURE 3-5

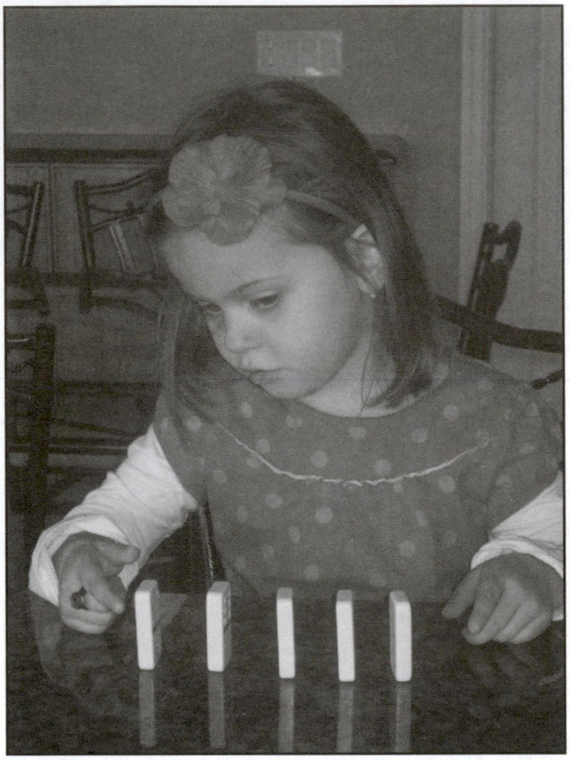

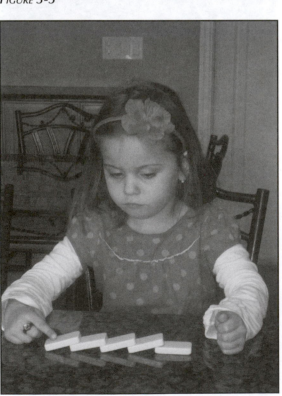

FIGURE 3-7

FIGURE 3-6

✦ Card stacking: Child copies different card-stacking houses from a model.

⬥ An easier version of this activity is building "houses" or pyramids by stacking disposable plastic cups.

✦ "Mummy wrapping game": Child wraps another child or adult with toilet paper. Child must use only light pressure when playing this game or else the toilet paper will rip. (Try to use heavy duty toilet paper for this project.)

✦ Bowling pins: Child sets up bowling pins or another light object flat on the floor or makes a tower with them. Child then crashes into it or rolls a ball into it.

✦ Yo-Yos: Therapist teaches child how to play with a yo-yo.

✦ Keyboard typing: Child types different words or plays different games on a computer keyboard.

✦ Lining up figurines: Child lines up small figurines gently, trying not to let them fall.

COMMERCIALLY AVAILABLE PRODUCTS

✦ "Penguin Pile-Up"
✦ "Barrel of Monkeys"
✦ "Pick Up Sticks"
✦ "Kerplunk"
✦ "Don't Break the Ice"
✦ "Don't Spill the Beans"
✦ "Super Catch"
✦ "Jenga"
✦ "Topple"

BILATERAL INTEGRATION/ CROSSING MIDLINE

Bilateral integration is the ability to coordinate both sides of the body for a purposeful action. There are different components to bilateral integration. Bilateral integration includes performing an act with both sides of the body simultaneously. This is called *symmetrical bilateral integration* (e.g., rolling playdough with a rolling pin, clapping hands, etc.). It also refers to using both sides of the body *reciprocally*, as in alternating movements (e.g., climbing stairs). Finally, bilateral integration includes using each side of the body for a different action simultaneously. This is called *asymmetrical bilateral integration (e.g.,* stabilizing a paper with one hand while writing with the other, or holding a jar with one hand while unscrewing the cover with the other).

Crossing midline: *Midline* is a vertical line down the middle of one's body. Crossing midline means using a body part, such as the hand or foot, to reach across the midline of the body. An example of crossing midline would be reaching for a puzzle piece with one's right hand when the piece is placed on the left side of one's body. The left side of the brain controls the right side of the body and the right side of the brain controls the left side of the body. Crossing midline requires integrating and using both sides of the brain together. It is more challenging to use both sides of the brain simultaneously and, therefore, this is often difficult for many children.

Bilateral integration and crossing midline support a child's development of fine motor skills, academic skills, and functional skills. It is needed for many everyday activities, such as dressing (i.e., putting on socks, driving a car [e.g., turning the steering wheel], writing [e.g., writing across a page], and many play activities) (Van Hof, Van Der Kamp, & Savelsbergh, 2002).

In order to be able to cross midline, one needs adequate bilateral integration skills. Many activities that involve crossing midline also require the use of both hands and sides of the body simultaneously. One could say that bilateral integration and crossing midline "go hand in hand." It is for this reason that crossing midline and bilateral integration activities were put into the same section.

When working with a child with poor bilateral integration skills, it is important to be aware of ways children will compensate for this deficit. Although a child may show a right-hand preference, this child will reach for objects on his/her left side with the left hand and transfer the object into the right hand in order to avoid crossing midline.

When setting up a therapeutic activity, it can be helpful to remind the child to use the dominant hand to pick up objects, regardless of the location of the object (i.e., whether the object is to the left or right of the child). This will help remind the child to cross midline. Many children will still avoid crossing midline by moving the direction of their trunk in order to face the object. It is important to help a child stabilize the trunk when reaching, thereby forcing the child to cross midline.

Danto, A., & Pruzansky, M. *1001 Pediatric Treatment Activities: Creative Ideas for Therapy Sessions* (pp. 35-44).
© 2011 SLACK Incorporated

Bilateral Integration/Crossing Midline Treatment Activities

Symmetrical Bilateral Integration

+ Legos: Child plays with Legos, pushing together pieces and pulling them apart.
+ Playdough: Child plays with playdough, rolls it, flattens it, makes a ball with it, and uses playdough toys and accessories.
+ Theraputty: Child pulls and pushes Theraputty.
+ Child pushes together/pulls apart toys—e.g., pegs or pop beads.
+ Child opens and closes plastic eggs (Figure 4-1).

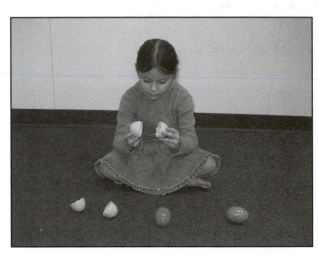

FIGURE *4-1*

+ Snow baller: Child uses a snow baller to pick toys off of floor (Figures 4-2 and 4-3).
  ⬦ Upgrade this activity by having child on a balance beam or on suspended equipment when using the snow baller to pick up the toys.

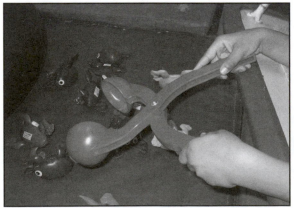

FIGURE *4-2*

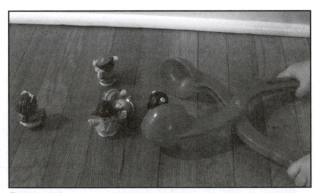

FIGURE *4-3*

✦ Dribbling games: Child dribbles a basketball in each hand at the same time (Figure 4-4).

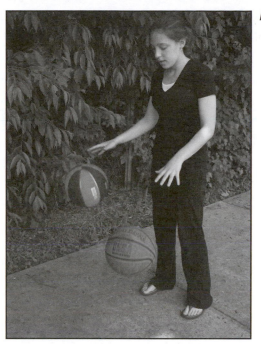

FIGURE 4-4

✦ Rapper Snappers: Child pulls apart/pushes together accordion plastics (Figures 4-5 and 4-6).

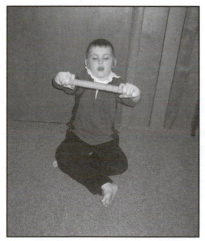

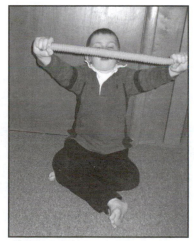

FIGURE 4-5

FIGURE 4-6

Crossing Midline

In order to help children become more aware of their midlines, while practicing crossing midline activities, place painters tape in a vertical line on the midline of the trunk.

✦ Children's clapping games: Child #1 faces child #2. Both children claps hands together then clap alternate hand on opposite child (child #1's right hand hits child #2's right hand), and then repeats with other hand. Some games include:

   ✧ Miss Mary Mack.
   ✧ Patty Cake (Figure 4-7).

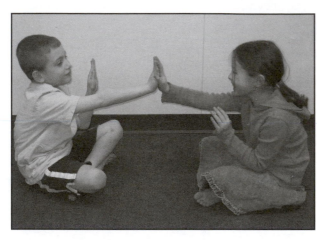

FIGURE 4-7

✦ Cheerleading games: Therapist gives child pom-poms and has child watch therapist in order to imitate various cheers. Cheers should include crossing midline and using both arms together (Figures 4-8 and 4-9).

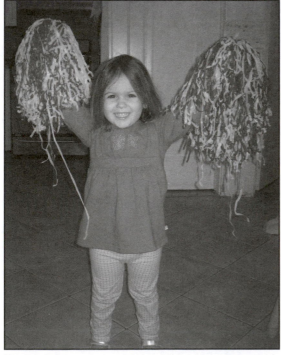

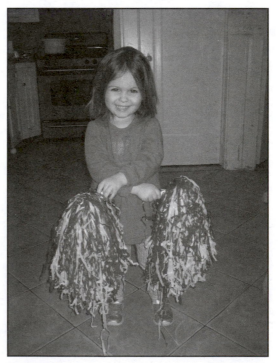

FIGURE 4-8

FIGURE 4-9

- Stretching:
    - Child stands up and brings one hand to opposite foot and switches. Repeat as tolerated.
    - Child sits in a chair and brings one elbow to the opposite knee and then switches and repeats activity as tolerated.
- Figure 8's:
    - Therapist tapes a large figure 8 on floor. Child walks in a figure 8-style over tape.
    - Child traces small, horizontal figure 8's on a piece of paper.
    - Child traces large, horizontal figure 8's on a chalkboard and continues going around the figure 8 several times.
- Therapist places balance beam on floor. Child walks crisscrossing legs over the balance beam when walking along.
- Child holds a basketball and moves it in a circle around stomach, back, and back to the front (Figure 4-10).

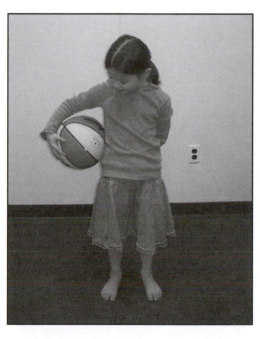

FIGURE 4-10

- Child pretends to drive a car, using a ball as the steering wheel. Therapist encourages child to cross hand over hand when turning the steering wheel (Figure 4-11).

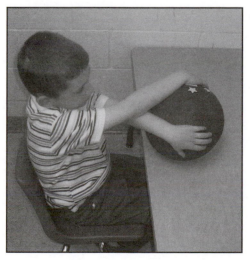

FIGURE 4-11

+ Dancing activities:
    ✧ Therapist puts on music with a marching beat. Child marches around room with right knee touching left elbow and left knee touching right elbow.
    ✧ Child dances with scarves, making figure 8's with arms while waving the scarves.
+ Therapist places child in supine on playmat with hanging toys. Encourage young child (developmental age of 3 to 9 months approximately) to swat/reach for toys on both sides (Figure 4-12).

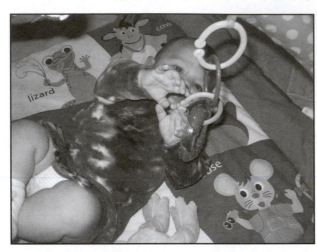

Figure 4-12

+ Place child in upright sitting position with toys placed within reach of child on both sides. Encourage child to reach for toys on both sides (Figure 4-13).

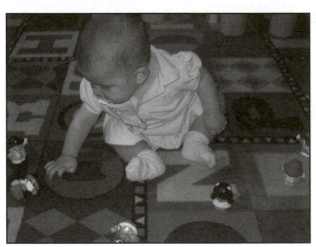

Figure 4-13

Reciprocal Hand Use

◆ Child performs jumping jacks.

◆ Bicycle sit-ups: Child lies on back and brings the right elbow to the left knee, while extending the right leg. Then switches and repeats as tolerated (Figure 4-14).

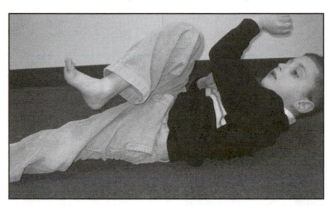

FIGURE 4-14

◆ Climbing: Child climbs up a ladder or climbs up a flight of stairs on his/her hands.

◆ Double-Dutch jump rope: Child tries to swing two jump ropes at a time in the "Double-Dutch" style.

◆ Juggling: Therapist teaches child how to juggle two or more balls (Figure 4-15). Juggling with scarves or weighted bean bags may be a little easier than balls.

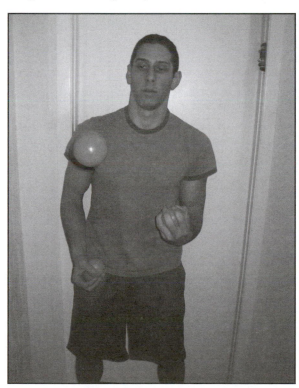

FIGURE 4-15

Asymmetrical Bilateral Integration

✦ Lacing beads: Child holds string in one hand and a bead in the other. Child uses both hands to lace bead onto string.

✦ Child opens and closes jars.

✦ Child screws and unscrews nuts and bolts.

✦ Cutting activities: Child cuts strips of paper, shapes, or diagrams. (See Appendix pp. 213-222 for sample cutting activities.)

✦ Paper ring project: Child cuts out multiple strips of paper. Child glues the ends of one strip together to make a ring. Child then loops the additional strips of paper, one at a time, around the initial ring to add on more rings. Child glues the ends together, and keeps adding more rings to make a chain of paper rings (Figure 4-16).

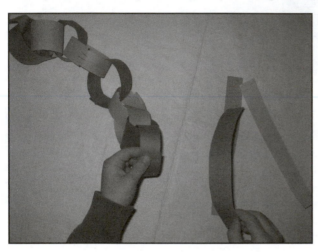

FIGURE 4-16

✦ Lacing cards: Child uses lacing cards to lace a string in and out of the holes with one hand while stabilizing the lacing card with the other hand. (Lacing cards/boards can be created by laminating a small piece of construction paper and punching holes approximately 1 inch apart around the perimeter of the laminated paper.)

✦ Therapist gives child a sandwich cookie for a snack to break open in halves.

✦ Braiding: Child practices braiding on either hair, on dolls, or with pipe cleaners.

✦ Caterpillar toy: Pull rings off/put rings on (Figure 4-17).

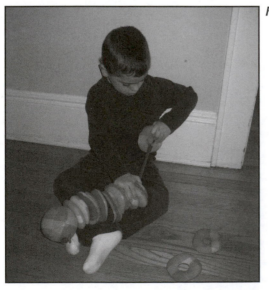

FIGURE 4-17

◆ Paper airplane making: Therapist teaches child how to make paper airplanes. Therapist performs each step separately and slowly. After each step therapist waits until child is caught up. Therapist assists child to ensure the folding is performed accurately.

◆ Table tapping: Therapist sits facing child and places both his/her hands and the child's hands on the desk. One person starts by tapping the desk once with one hand. The four hands on the desk surface should try and tap the desk, one hand at a time, in a clockwise fashion. If someone taps twice in a row quickly, that alternates the direction of the circle to counterclockwise (Figure 4-18).

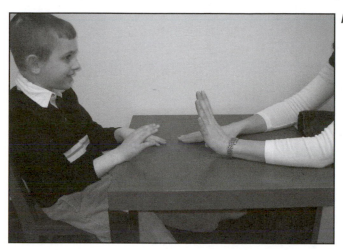

FIGURE 4-18

◆ Hoop jumping: Therapist places different colored hoops on the floor (Figure 4-19). Child alternates stepping into each hoop with feet and calls out the color of the hoop as the foot steps down into it. In order to upgrade this activity, place pictures of different letters inside the hoops and have child call out the letter in the hoop (Figure 4-20). Place pictures of animals in the hoops and have child call out name of animal (Figure 4-21).

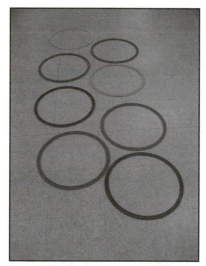
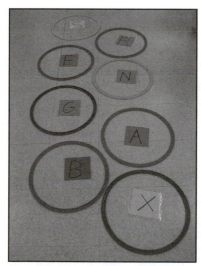
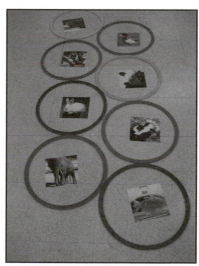

FIGURE 4-19   *FIGURE 4-20*   *FIGURE 4-21*

+ Knitting activities (Figure 4-22).

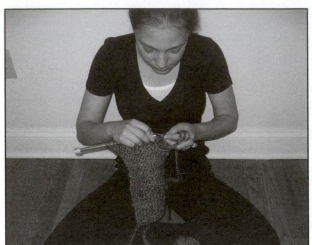

FIGURE 4-22

COMMERCIALLY AVAILABLE PRODUCTS

+ "Zoom Ball"
+ "Pop Beads"
+ "Kid K'nex"
+ "Mr. Potato Head"
+ "Velcro Fruit Game"
+ "Etch-a-Sketch"
+ "Smart Snacks Sorting Shapes Cupcakes"
+ "Oreo Matchin' Middles Game"
+ "Twister"

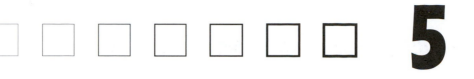

VESTIBULAR SYSTEM

The vestibular system controls a person's sense of movement, how one tolerates changes in movement, and the sense of balance. The vestibular system is controlled by small receptors in the ears, which send messages to the brain in order to interpret movement (Ayres, 2005, pp. 41-42). Therefore, changes in head position have a great impact on the vestibular system. Many children with sensory processing difficulties will have irregularities in their vestibular system. These children will either be over-responsive or under-responsive to movement.

A child that is over-responsive to movement may have what is called "gravitational insecurity." These children might fear movement and try to avoid having their feet off the ground in order to maintain a sense of stability. Some of the functional implications for increased sensitivity to movement include difficulties with climbing on playground equipment, riding in a car without becoming carsick, descending a flight of stairs, and playing on swings.

Children that are under-reactive to movement may act in different ways in order to provide themselves with increased movement. These types of children may constantly be running around, climbing on furniture, jumping off different surfaces, and may be unable to sit still in a classroom. These children are often mislabeled as having "behavioral" problems, when it is really a sensory processing disorder.

While there are many different theories about how to strengthen and regulate the vestibular system, the suggestions in this chapter provide activities that involve slow, controlled movement as well as fast-paced movement. It is up to the treating therapist to determine the appropriate speed and type of movement provided, based on the individual child's needs and vestibular system.

While this does not hold true to all children, the following basic principles of the vestibular system should be reviewed before completing any vestibular activities:

✦ Speed of movement: Different children will respond differently to different speeds of movement. While fast movement may be more intense for some children, slow movement can be just as powerful and intense depending on the child and how an activity is set up (Ayres, 2005, p. 42).

✦ Length of time: The longer a child is engaged in a vestibular activity, the more intense the input will be.

✦ Having a child close his/her eyes increases the intensity of the movement provided.

✦ Rotary movement (spinning) can be more intense, arousing, and stimulating.

✦ Linear movement (back and forth) may create a more calming and organizing effect.

✦ A child's physical position will affect the intensity of the input. Having a child sit upright is less intense than laying a child on the back or side (Ayres, 2005, p. 42).

> *It is important to look for signs of nausea and dizziness when engaging in movement activities. If a child becomes nauseous during an activity, stop immediately. It may also help to follow up with a proprioceptive activity in the form of deep pressure. This may help provide the child with a grounding feeling and decrease the level of nausea. (It is ideal to avoid having the child reach the point of nausea.)*

> **Before selecting or implementing any movement activities, it is important to first review these ideas with an occupational therapist.**

Danto, A., & Pruzansky, M. *1001 Pediatric Treatment Activities: Creative Ideas for Therapy Sessions* (pp. 45-52). © 2011 SLACK Incorporated

Activities To Strengthen Vestibular System

Swinging

+ Child goes on different suspended equipment and swings: Allow child to place feet on floor at first, then attempt to swing child with feet off the floor.
+ Child swings on an outdoor hammock.
+ Child swings on a swing set swing (Figure 5-1).

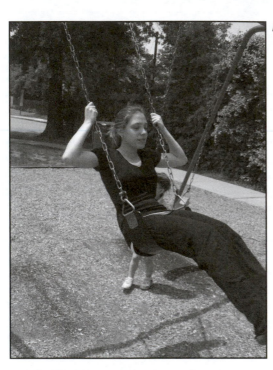

FIGURE 5-1

Changing Head Positions

+ Therapist slowly moves child's head in different planes of movement including to the side, backward, and forward.
+ Child bends down and looks under legs and waves hello to therapist.
+ Child bends down and throws a ball between legs to therapist (Figure 5-2).

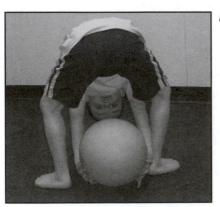

FIGURE 5-2

Slow, Controlled Movement

✦ Therapist slowly rocks child in different planes on rocker chair.

✦ Child slowly walks up and down ramp.

✦ Musical chairs: Child walks around a set of chairs and when the music stops, the child has to sit down in one of the chairs.

✦ Balance beam activities:

  ◇ Child walks across a balance beam backward and forward.

  ◇ Child walks across with eyes closed.

✦ Balance board activities:

  ◇ Child bends down to pick up toys off floor, then throws toys into a container/basket (Figure 5-3).

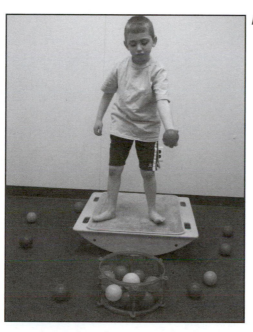

FIGURE 5-3

  ◇ Child steps up onto balance board.

  ◇ Child makes a 360-degree turn in place while standing on balance board.

  ◇ Child slaps hands with therapist in different directional planes (Figure 5-4).

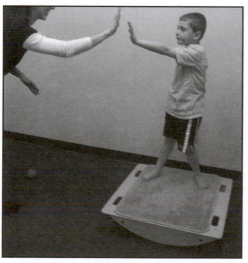

FIGURE 5-4

✧ Child pops bubbles all around (Figure 5-5).

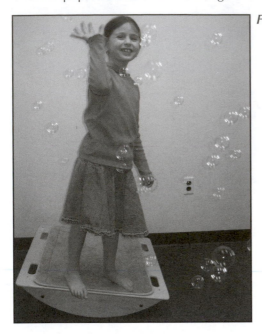

FIGURE 5-5

    ✧ Child plays catch.

    ✧ Child shoots basketballs.

    ✧ Child bends down to the floor and picks up objects.

✦ Child slowly walks up and down a flight of stairs, alternating feet when descending (instead of step-to-step pattern). Subsequently, child attempts to do this without holding onto the railing.

✦ "Roly-Poly Game": Child lies on a mat and slowly rolls from one end to the other. This can be made into a game with a group of children. Designate one child as the leader who determines in which direction to roll, when to start, and when to stop. The object of the game is to not bump into anyone else on the mat.

✦ Child goes inside a barrel. Therapist slowly rolls child on the floor across the room.

✦ Child sits on a swivel chair and is slowly spun around in both directions.

✦ Child climbs over big pillows and bolsters or any uneven surface.

✦ Child walks up onto a cube chair and then slowly steps down (Figure 5-6). (Child can alternatively jump down.)

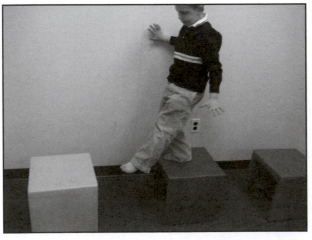

FIGURE 5-6

✦ "Ring Around the Rosie": Children hold hands with therapist or other children and slowly move around in a circle singing "Ring Around the Rosie."

✦ Chair rides: Child sits on a chair with wheels. Therapist slowly pulls the child around room on chair.

✦ Somersaults: Child performs somersaults on a mat on the floor.

✦ Child sits on "Dizzy Disc" with legs crossed and is spun around or child can lie on belly on dizzy disc and spin self around in circles (Figures 5-7 and 5-8).

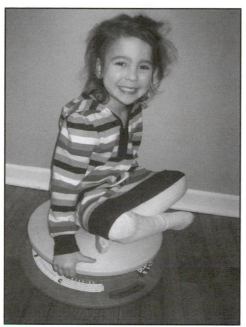
FIGURE 5-7

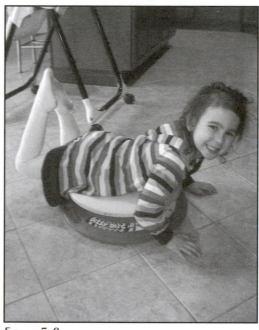
FIGURE 5-8

Fast-Paced Input

✦ Therapy ball:
  ◇ Therapist bounces child on the ball and then tips the child from side to side.
  ◇ Therapist places child in prone position (on the belly) on the ball and then tips the child forward and to sides (Figure 5-9).

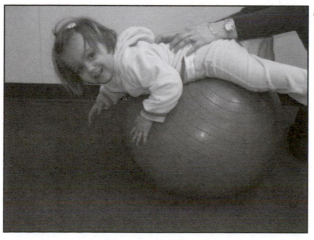
FIGURE 5-9

✦ Hippity Hop: Child bounces across the room on a Hippity Hop toy (Figure 5-10).

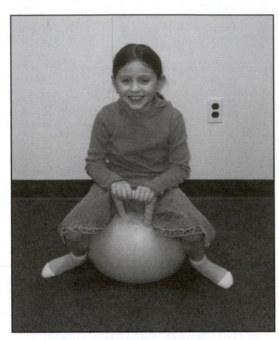

FIGURE 5-10

✦ Child slides down slides of varying heights and turns.

✦ Two children go on a seesaw, one at each end. Children alternate between going up and down.

✦ Child sits on a scooter while being spun around several times by therapist as tolerated.

✦ Trampoline games:

   ⬥ Child jumps on a trampoline and counts to ten.

   ⬥ Child runs in place on the trampoline.

   ⬥ Child sits on the trampoline and tries to bounce up and down by moving body to create momentum.

✦ Tag: Child plays "tag" or another fast-moving chasing game.

✦ Jumping off surfaces of varying heights: Child holds hands with therapist and jumps in the air off of the floor. Child then jumps off a slightly higher surface. Therapist should continue raising the height of the surface slightly. If at any point the child is fearful, allow child to hold both of the therapist's hands or fingers. Provide child with as minimal physical assistance as possible.

✦ Child quickly walks up and down a flight of stairs, alternating feet when descending (instead of step-to-step pattern). Subsequently, child attempts to do this without holding onto the railing.

✦ Child sits on a swivel chair and is quickly spun around in both directions.

✦ Chair rides: Child sits on a chair with wheels. Therapist quickly pulls child around the room on chair.

✦ Child rocks back and forth on rocking playground toys (Figure 5-11).

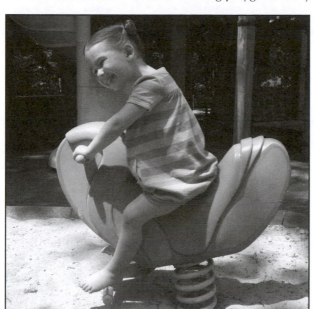

FIGURE 5-11

TACTILE SENSITIVITY

Tactile sensitivity and tactile defensiveness are conditions in which a child finds different types of touch aversive. This occurs because the touch receptors in the child's skin are hypersensitive to different forms of touch. A child with tactile sensitivity usually has specific fibers, materials, and foods that he/she will not tolerate (Ayres, 2005, p. 105). One first must identify these factors before working with the child. It is also important to distinguish true tactile defensiveness from other behavioral and medical problems.

There are many exercises and activities that can be done in order to help decrease tactile sensitivity. Light touch is usually more uncomfortable to a child with tactile sensitivity, versus deep pressure touch. When performing the activities in this section, it is important to grade these activities by presenting the child with the least noxious stimuli and gradually introducing more noxious stimuli. This is to ensure that the child does not become overly stressed.

Danto, A., & Pruzansky, M. *1001 Pediatric Treatment Activities:*
Creative Ideas for Therapy Sessions (pp. 53-56).
© 2011 SLACK Incorporated

Activities To Decrease Tactile Sensitivity

Deep Pressure

+ Lotion massage: Therapist massages child's hand with lotion, applying firm and consistent pressure.
+ Squishy toys: Child squeezes and releases toys with different squishy textures.
+ Wheelbarrow walking: Child wheelbarrow walks across the room.
+ While lying prone on a scooter board, child propels self around the room using the palms of his hands.
+ Playdough: Child plays with playdough, rolling it, and squeezing it with both hands.
+ Brushing protocol: refer to Pat Willbarger's brushing protocol (Wilbarger & Wilbarger, 1991).

Becoming Comfortable With an Outside Touch

+ Graded exposure to textures: Child rubs different textured fabrics and toys on back and front of the hand as tolerated. Child also attempts this activity with eyes closed and sees if it is possible to identify the objects placed in child's hand without the assistance of vision.
+ Child strokes the back and front of the hand with a feather.
+ Vibrating massage: Child uses a vibrating toy or massager to massage both hands. Child massages both the front and back of the hand as tolerated.
+ Vibrating toothbrush: Child brushes teeth with a vibrating tooth brush.
+ Therapist plays "This little piggy…" on the child's fingers (Figure 6-1).

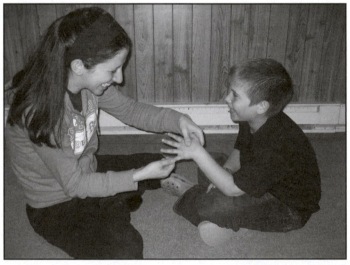

Figure 6-1

+ Face painting: Therapist applies face paint to child's face and cheeks. If child will not tolerate this, allow child to apply the face paint to own face directly.
+ Touching faces: Therapist uses fingers to touch different parts of child's face and neck as tolerated by child.

Grainy Textures

+ Sandbox activities: Child plays in sandbox and makes small castles with sand or finds hidden objects in sand. Additionally, child can make different shapes and spell different letters in sand.

✦ Child finds hidden objects in a rice box or bag full of beans (Figure 6-2).

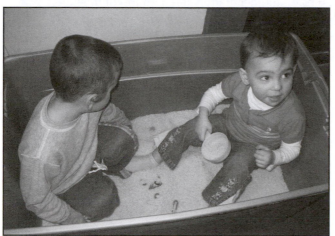

FIGURE 6-2

✦ Sandpaper project: Child assists in smoothing rough wood.
  Be careful of splinters.

✦ Child crunches up pieces of Corn Flakes (or another crunchy cereal) with his/her hands and sprinkles them onto a piece of paper with glue to make a project.

Creamy and Wet Textures

✦ Shaving cream activity: Child spreads shaving cream on an inflated balloon. Child then uses his/her index finger to spell his/her name in the shaving cream or make a smiley face.

✦ Finger paint: Child engages in any finger painting projects including making pictures, shapes, and spelling words in the paint.

✦ Hand-Tree project: Therapist places brown paint on child's forearm and hand. Child presses hand onto a white piece of paper. This will provide a tree trunk and branches. Therapist then places different colored paint on child's fingertips and has child press down on the tree branches to make leaves and fruit (Figures 6-3 through 6-5).

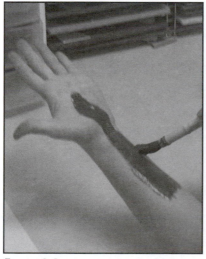
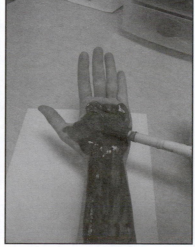
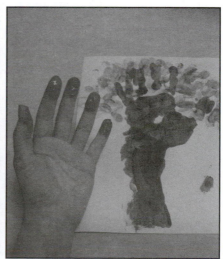

FIGURE 6-3   *FIGURE 6-4*   *FIGURE 6-5*

+ Sticky glue project: Child uses colored or regular glue to squeeze on a piece of paper and then spreads it out with index finger. Child can then place sequins or another craft material on top of the glue.

+ Marshmallow Fluff project: Child makes a Marshmallow Fluff sandwich. Child spreads fluff on a piece of bread or cracker with fingers. Allow child to place some toppings onto the fluff (raisins, sprinkles, pretzels, chips, etc.).

+ Child spreads peanut butter on a plastic plate—enough to cover the whole surface. Child then spreads chocolate pudding on top of the peanut butter. Child traces different letters on the plate. Allow child to lick finger after each letter.

> *Be sure to first check for food allergies.*

+ Water play: Child plays with water in a sink, pouring water from one container to another and then onto his/her hands. Therapist should vary the temperature of the water from warm to cool. Child should then squeeze washcloths and sponges.

> *Be sure to supervise this activity to make sure that the water temperature does not become dangerously hot.*

+ Water hunt: Therapist blindfolds child and has child pick out certain objects from the water.

> *Therapist must use sound judgment when selecting blindfolding activity with a specific child and must carefully supervise any activity involving blindfolding.*

+ Kneading activities: Child kneads bread or cookie dough to make a baking project.

+ Silly Putty: Child pulls Silly Putty and presses it onto different surfaces.

+ Playdough: Child rolls and pinches playdough.

+ Papier-Mâché piñata: Child dips strips of newspaper into papier-mâché flour/water mixture and places them on an inflated balloon. Child covers the entire surface except a small opening at the top. Let newspaper harden for a day, cut a small opening in the top, and then paint balloon and place candy inside.

+ Juice making: Child squeezes oranges or grapes into a cup to make fresh juice.

COMMERCIALLY AVAILABLE PRODUCTS

+ "Image Captor"
+ "Guidecraft Feel & Find Game"
+ "Moon Sand"
+ "Floam"

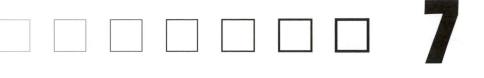

ORAL MOTOR

Oral motor exercises consist of activities that require the use of the tongue, mouth, lips, and surrounding facial muscles. These exercises can be helpful with feeding, speech and language, drooling problems, arousal level, and attention. The purpose of oral motor exercises can be either to strengthen, stimulate, or increase oral motor awareness.

These activities can be performed in preparation for another activity or as an activity in itself. It is important to watch for signs of fatigue when a child is performing these exercises. If the child has feeding/swallowing difficulties, it is important to first check with a doctor or speech therapist before attempting these activities. Additionally, when working on oral motor issues, the treating therapist should always first check for any dental problems or whether the child has a strong bite reflex. It is also important not to place small objects in a child's mouth who may have a tendency to eat nonfood objects.

Danto, A., & Pruzansky, M. *1001 Pediatric Treatment Activities:
Creative Ideas for Therapy Sessions* (pp. 57-62).
© 2011 SLACK Incorporated

Oral Motor Exercises

Increasing Lip Closure and Cheek Strength

+ Child blows bubbles on a bubble wand or bubble stick.
+ Child sticks a straw into a cup or bowl with water and blows down to create bubbles.
+ Child plays with blower toys (Figure 7-1).

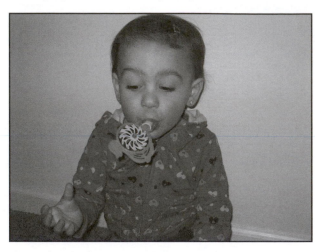

FIGURE 7-1

+ Child blows whistles and kazoos.
+ Therapist teaches child how to play a song on a recorder or has child make fun noises with the recorder.
+ Child blows pom-poms or cotton balls across a table (Figure 7-2).

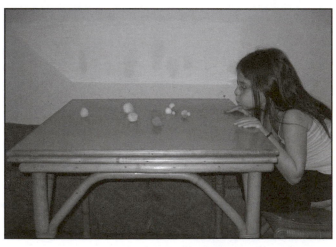

FIGURE 7-2

+ Therapist cuts out a paper fish and place it on a table. Child then blows it into a specific target (e.g., into a bucket with water).

✦ Therapist tapes a small piece of paper or a feather to the end of a straw and has child blow (Figure 7-3).

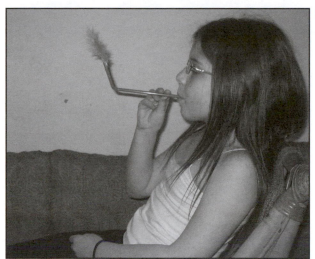

FIGURE 7-3

Sound Making

✦ Therapist babbles and attempts to get child to imitate.

✦ Therapist makes different sounds and noises and attempts to get child to imitate.

✦ Therapist and child sing a song with many different sounds. For example, sing "Witch Doctor" song ("Ooo eee ooo ah ah") or "Old McDonald Had a Farm ("Ee i ee i oh") in order to practice making different sounds in fun way.

Exercises for Overall Strengthening of Oral Structures

✦ Jaw strengthening exercises: Child bites down on Popsicle stick while therapist pulls on it or child places a Popsicle stick horizontally in mouth and bites down using teeth (Figures 7-4 and 7-5).

   Therapist should first check for any dental problems with child or for issues with bite reflexes.

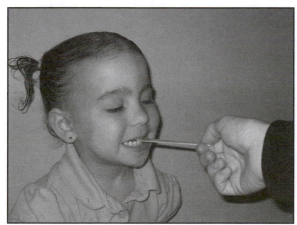

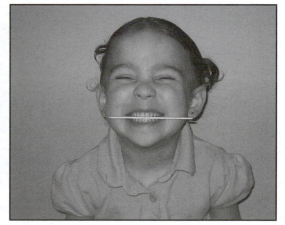

FIGURE 7-4   *FIGURE 7-5*

✦ Lip-strengthening exercises: Therapist places a Popsicle stick between child's lips and has child hold this position (Figure 7-6).

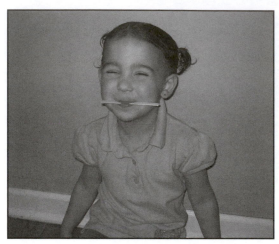

FIGURE 7-6

✦ Tongue tug-of-war: Therapist wraps gauze around child's tongue and gently pulls it out of child's mouth. Have child try and resist this.

✦ Cheek thrusts: Child sticks out tongue into the side of the mouth in order to make one cheek stick out. Therapist pushes against the side of child's cheek trying to push against the tongue.

✦ Tongue push-ups: Child places a Cheerio, M&M, or a Froot Loop on the top of the mouth and pushes tongue up against if for a couple seconds at a time, gradually increasing the amount of time the tongue can stay pushed to the top of the mouth.

✦ Gum chewing: Therapist places gum on the child's back molars and has child practice biting up and down, gradually increasing amount of times he/she can bite down (Rosenfeld-Johnson, 2001, p. 110-117 [Review Rosenfeld-Johnson reference for sample gum-chewing protocol.]).

✦ Child sucks liquids through a crazy straw. Therapist should vary the thickness and texture of the liquids.

✦ Therapist places jelly/Marshmallow Fluff/peanut butter on the roof of child's mouth and has child lick it off.

✦ Therapist places jelly/Marshmallow Fluff/peanut butter on the top lip and has child lick it off (Figure 7-7).

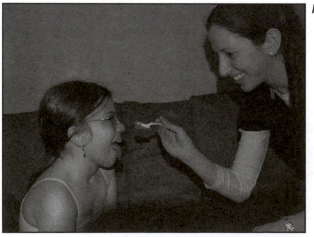

FIGURE 7-7

✦ Therapist provides child with crunchy and sticky foods to chew.

✦ Child copies tongue movements and positions, including up, down, side-to-side, and all around.

✦ Child copies lip positions, including purse, pucker, smile, frown, open, and close.

✦ Tongue scavenger hunt: Therapist touches child's lips and skin around the mouth, or any spot inside the mouth with either a tongue depressor or a lollipop. Child then must point to the spot touched with the tip of the tongue.

✦ Fish face: Child tries to imitate a "fish face," holds the position for several seconds, and then relaxes facial muscles. Repeat as tolerated (Figure 7-8).

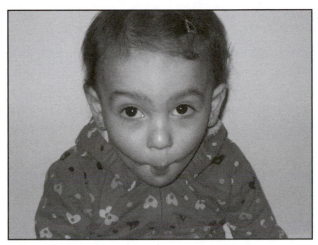

FIGURE 7-8

✦ Therapist places a small amount of Chapstick on child's lips and has child try to spread the Chapstick onto the entire surface of the lips without using hands.

Stimulating the Mouth Through Sensory Input

✦ Therapist provides compression to child's back molars.

✦ Therapist touches and massages different parts of child's face with a warm and cold wet cloth in order to expose the face to different temperatures.

✦ Therapist gently taps the skin around the child's mouth and has the child do the same.

✦ Child places Z-Vibe toy in mouth.

✦ Therapist stimulates different areas in and around the mouth with a "Nuk" brush (Figures 7-9 and 7-10).

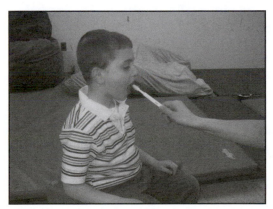

FIGURE 7-9

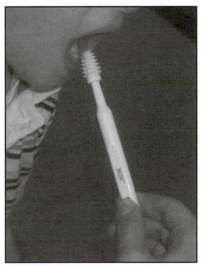

FIGURE 7-10

+ Therapist massages different parts of child's face and surrounding area with lotion.
+ Plain facial and lip massage: Therapist gently massages the skin around the child's mouth and the lips as tolerated.
+ Ark Grabbers/Chewy Tubes: Child bites down and releases on chewy toy (Figure 7-11).

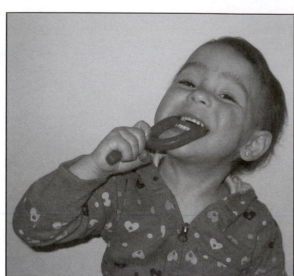

FIGURE 7-11

VISUAL SYSTEM

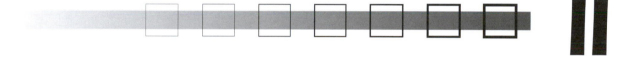

II

The visual system is an important system the body uses to give information about what one sees in the environment. There are many different components to the visual system that affect one's vision. These components will be discussed further in the upcoming chapters.

This section focuses on three main components of the visual system: visual perception, visual motor integration, and visual scanning. It then provides useful activities that can help strengthen each system individually.

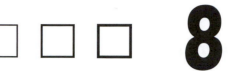

VISUAL PERCEPTION

Visual perception is how the eyes interpret what one sees into meaningful information. There are many different components to visual perception. Some of these areas include visual discrimination (the ability to discriminate between two similar forms), visual form constancy (the ability to recognize the same form when it appears in a different way), visual figure ground (the ability to find a form when it is hidden among other forms), visual closure (the ability to recognize a form when the complete form is not visible), visual spatial relations (the ability to determine the correct direction of forms), and visual memory (the ability to remember the details of a single form) (Martin, 2006).

A child with poor visual perceptual skills will be affected in many ways, academically and functionally. Visual perception affects one's ability to complete puzzles, write neatly on paper, learn how to recognize letters and numbers, find a toy on a messy shelf, and complete any sorting task.

This chapter will provide different visual perceptual exercises that can help strengthen the visual perceptual system through fun games and activities.

Danto, A., & Pruzansky, M. *1001 Pediatric Treatment Activities:*
Creative Ideas for Therapy Sessions (pp. 65-72).
© 2011 SLACK Incorporated

Visual Perceptual Activities

Visual Discrimination

+ Child completes "What's Missing/What's Different Pictures." (See Appendix pp. 223-224 for sample pictures.)
+ Therapist shows child a string of four different pictures and asks child to figure out which two pictures are exactly alike and circle them. (See Appendix pp. 225-227 for sample pictures.)
+ Dot marker game: Therapist takes different colored markers and makes big and small scattered circles on a page with the different colors. Child should then be given dot markers and be told to place the corresponding colored dot into each circle on the page (Figure 8-1). (See Appendix p. 228 for sample dot marker handout.)

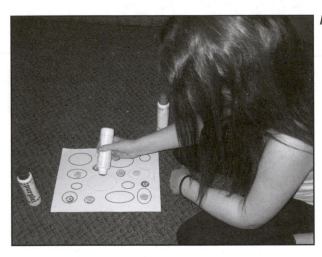

FIGURE 8-1

+ Verbal descriptions: When learning how to write new letters, therapist has child verbally describe the letter. This may help the child remember the different attributes of a letter and be able to write and recognize it more easily.
+ Sorting games:
  ⬥ Puzzle piece sorting: Child assists in sorting center puzzle pieces from edge puzzle pieces.
  ⬥ Child plays with color and shape sorters.
  ⬥ Baseball card sorting: Child sorts players by team, league, etc.
  ⬥ Deck of cards: Child sorts cards by suit, number, etc.
  ⬥ Froot Loops sorting activity: Therapist places Froot Loops all over table and gives child five strings. Child makes five different necklaces that are all one specific color.
+ Copy patterns:
  ⬥ Froot Loops necklaces: Therapist places different colored Froot Loops on a string to make a necklace. Child copies the pattern of colors on the original necklace. This activity can be upgraded or downgraded based on the complexity of the pattern and the amount of colors used in making the necklace (i.e., use anywhere from 2 to 6 colors when creating the original pattern).

✧ Peg patterns: Child places pegs into a peg board in a specific order, copying a set pattern (Figure 8-2).

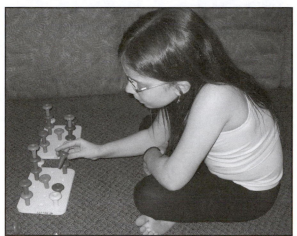

FIGURE 8-2

✧ Necklace making: Therapist provides child with different colored beads and has child copy a pattern with the beads.

Visual Form Constancy

✦ Ball bouncing game
   ✧ Part I: Therapist places different random letters on the wall and asks child to spell a word by throwing a ball against the letters, one at a time, in the correct order in order to spell the word.
   ✧ Part II: Child covers eyes while therapist flips the letters on the wall so the letters are upside down, sideways or backward. Child opens eyes to look at the letters and tries and spell the same word.
✦ Letter recognition: Therapist writes the letters of the alphabet in different ways on multiple index cards or pieces of paper. For example therapist can write the letter "A" in a big size, little size, uppercase, lowercase, cursive, red, blue, and yellow. Therapist should do this for several more letters, mix the letters up, and scatter them on the floor. Child should then try and find all of the different "A"s hidden on the floor and subsequently the other letters as well.
✦ View Appendix pp. 229-230 for form constancy handout.

Visual Figure Ground

✦ Hidden pictures: Child finds different hidden objects in a picture. (See Appendix pp. 231-232 for sample hidden picture handout.)
✦ Child completes "Word Searches/Word Finds."
✦ Finding objects in a competing background: Child finds a specific toy either somewhere in the room or on a messy shelf among other toys.
✦ Therapist places laminated letters all around floor and has child jump over, hop over, or touch the letters of child's name.
✦ "I Spy": Therapist should look around the room and think of an object in the room. Therapist should give clues about the object (e.g., size, color, specific features). Child has to look around the room to find it. Child is allowed to ask for hints and other clues.
✦ "Find the Letter": Child copies a word, sentence, or paragraph onto a piece of paper. Therapist provides child with a red pen or marker. Child then goes back to composition and looks for a specific letter. For example, choose the letter "R." Have the child read over the written work and circle all of the "R's" on the page.

✦ Some compensatory strategies to help a child with poor figure ground skills include:

⬥ Limit visual distractions by keeping a child's work area free of clutter.

⬥ Have child sit in the front of the classroom to limit visual distractions.

⬥ When providing a written assignment for the child, write as little on every page as possible. For example, for a math homework assignment, write only one math problem on each page.

⬥ Use bright and colorful borders around the paper the child is writing on to give an additional visual cue. Some children might find this distracting and may benefit more from a dark black border around the paper they are working on.

Visual Closure

✦ Puzzles: Child completes different puzzles.

⬥ The easiest type of puzzle is a form puzzle (Figure 8-3).

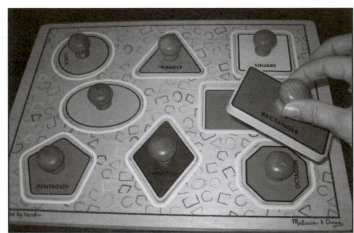

FIGURE 8-3

⬥ The next level of difficulty is a cut puzzle (Figure 8-4).

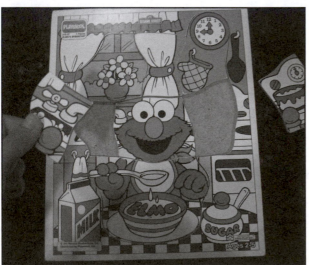

FIGURE 8-4

❖ The most challenging type of puzzle is an interlocking puzzle (Figure 8-5).

FIGURE 8-5

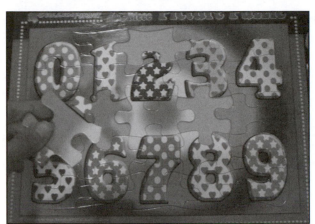

✦ Child completes interlocking puzzle with many small pieces (Figure 8-6).

FIGURE 8-6

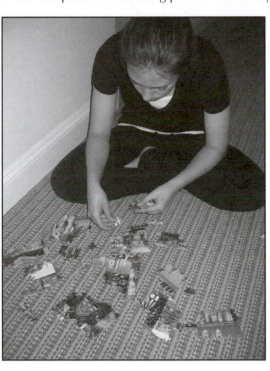

✦ When putting a puzzle together, therapist asks child to identify an object in a specific puzzle piece without looking at the completed puzzle picture.

✦ Incomplete puzzles: Therapist assists child in putting together a puzzle, but hides several pieces from the puzzle. Therapist asks child to identify what is the picture in the puzzle with only part of the puzzle completed.

✦ Letter identification: Therapist writes parts of a letter on a paper and has child try and identify which letter it is. (See Appendix p. 233 for sample handout.)

✦ Word identification: Therapist writes parts of the different letters in a word to see if the child is able to identify the word. This activity can also be played by covering the bottom quarter of a word with a piece of paper to see if the child can guess the word with only the top three quarters of the word visible. (See Appendix p. 234 for sample handout.)

✦ Picture identification: Therapist creates a picture and covers up part of it to see if child is able to identify the item in the picture (See Appendix pp. 235-236 for sample handout.)

Visual Spatial Relations

✦ Child completes "Shape/Size Sorter Worksheet" (See Appendix pp. 213-216 for handout.)

✦ Puzzles: Child assists in turning the puzzle pieces in the correct direction.

✦ Shape matching: Therapist cuts out four of same shape or picture. Therapist places the shapes on the table with one shape placed on the table above the other three. The three shapes should all be facing a different direction with only one of them placed in the same direction as the shape on top of the others. Child then identifies which shape matches the direction of the shape on top (Figure 8-7).

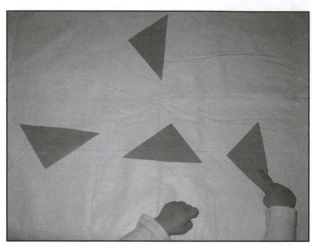

FIGURE 8-7

✦ Lego matching: This game is the same as the shape matching game (listed above), but played with Lego pieces. Therapist places four of the exact same Legos on the table. One of the Legos should be in a row of its own on top of the other three. The bottom three Legos should all face a different direction from each other, except one should face the same direction as the Lego on top. Child picks which Lego is facing the same direction as the one on top.

✦ Key holes: Therapist draws a picture of a pretend keyhole and picture of a pretend key. Therapist cuts out the key and asks child to turn the key in the correct direction needed to place the key into the hole.

✦ "SET": Child plays the game of SET with another child in order to find shapes/patterns with different orientations and colors (Figure 8-8).

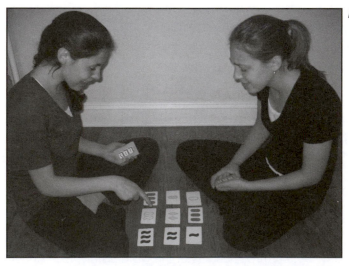

FIGURE 8-8

✦ "Oops letter writing": Therapist deliberately writes a letter on the board with an error (upside down, backward, etc.). Child tries to verbally describe the error with the letter.

+ "Be the teacher": Child copies a sentence or writes a composition on a piece of lined paper. Provide the child with a special felt-tipped marker or pen. Have the child go back and edit the paper, circling every letter that does not reach the line when it is supposed to, or letters that go below the line when they are not supposed to. Give the child one point for every correct circle and try to have the child reach a set score.

+ A child that has difficulty writing neatly in a confined space may be having difficulty with visual spatial relations. It may be helpful to use different types of paper when completing handwriting in order to help a child visualize the correct place on the paper to write. These papers include:

  ⬦ Graph paper: Child writes one letter per each slot on the graph paper (Figures 8-9 and 8-10). Use smaller or bigger boxed graph paper based on the child's handwriting level. The smaller the boxes, the more difficult the handwriting activity is.

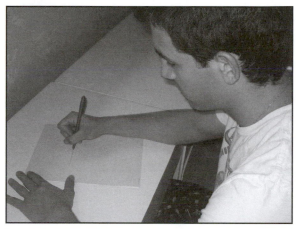

FIGURE 8-9

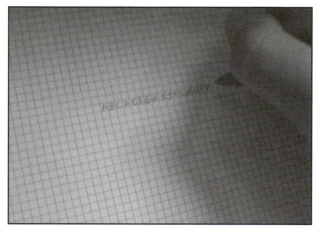

FIGURE 8-10

  ⬦ Raised line paper: This type of paper can help a child feel a physical boundary when writing.

  ⬦ Visual clues: Therapist colors over the margin line with a thick red marker in order to remind the child the starting place to come back to when the child finishes writing on a specific line.

  ⬦ Additional visual cues: A child that has difficulty organizing overall writing may require some other visual cue aside from the margin line. It may be helpful to place a sticker or a star in the upper left corner of the page to remind the child where writing starts. *Handwriting Without Tears* provides prefabricated paper like this.

Visual Memory

+ Memory/Concentration games: This can be played with an actual "Memory Game" or can be self-made. Therapist places pairs of cards face down on the table. Child flips over two cards at a time, trying to find a match.

+ Froot Loops memory game: Therapist shows the child a card with a sequence of colors written on it, for example: red, orange, yellow, blue. The card is then removed and the child makes a Froot Loops necklace with the correct order of colors.

+ "Busy picture" books: Child looks at a page on a "busy picture" book for a little while. The book is then closed and the child tells the therapist as many details about the page as possible.

Additional Visual Perceptual Resources

✦ Test of visual perceptual skills: Revised (TVPS-R)—The TVPS-R is meant to be used as an evaluation tool in order to test a child's visual perceptual skills. However, the different test items in this evaluation can be used in order to help a child practice and improve visual perceptual skills in the different areas of visual perception as well (Martin, 2006).

It is important to not use the TVPS-R to re-evaluate a child's visual perceptual skills if the child has practiced the different visual perceptual exercises on this test. Instead, another visual perceptual test can be used, including the Developmental Test of Visual Perception: Second Edition (DTVP-2) (Hammill, Pearson, & Voress, 1993).

On the Web

✦ Visit the following Web sites for additional visual perceptual activities:

  ✧ http://edhelper.com/visual_skills.htm

  ✧ www.eyecanlearn.com

COMMERCIALLY AVAILABLE PRODUCTS

- ✦ "Where's Waldo?"
- ✦ "Kid K'nex"
- ✦ "Perfection"
- ✦ "Dominoes"
- ✦ "Tic-Tac-Toe"
- ✦ "Magnetix"
- ✦ "Fantacolor Jr."
- ✦ "Checkers"
- ✦ "I Spy" board game
- ✦ "Picture Perfect Design Tiles"
- ✦ "Pattern Blocks & Board"
- ✦ "Design and Drill Activity Center"
- ✦ "Rush Hour Jr."
- ✦ "Katimino"
- ✦ "Lincoln Logs"
- ✦ "Oreo Matchin' Middles Game"
- ✦ "Smart Snacks Sorting Shapes Cupcakes"
- ✦ "Smart Snacks Mix & Match Doughnut Game"
- ✦ "Connect Four"
- ✦ "Tetris" computer game

VISUAL MOTOR INTEGRATION

Visual motor integration (VMI) is the ability of the eye to direct the hand and requires combined perceptual and motor skills. VMI skills affect a child's ability to write letters, copy figures, cut with scissors, complete mazes, stack blocks, and be successful in most sports activities.

When working on visual motor skills, it is important to identify which aspect of visual motor integration is difficult for the child (i.e., the motor component, the perceptual component, or both components are equally difficult). For example, a child that has difficulty completing mazes may struggle with moving a pencil within a confined space through the maze, but is able to easily see the correct path with his/her eyes. Conversely, another child may be able to easily guide a pencil through the same maze, but have difficulty visually locating the correct path to go along. Therefore, when selecting different visual motor exercises, it is important to identify which component of VMI is difficult for that particular child.

In this chapter, different VMI activities are provided. It is important to remember that VMI activities combine both perceptual and motor skills and one must keep this in mind when determining an appropriate choice of activity to challenge a child.

Danto, A., & Pruzansky, M. *1001 Pediatric Treatment Activities:*
Creative Ideas for Therapy Sessions (pp. 73-82).
© 2011 SLACK Incorporated

Visual Motor Activities

Cutting and Gluing

+ Cutting practice:
  ⬦ Child snips a narrow sheet of paper (Figure 9-1).

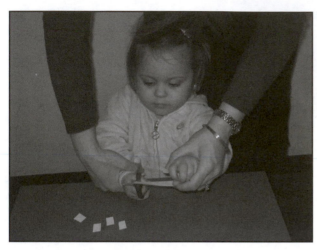

FIGURE 9-1

  ⬦ Child cuts on straight lines.
  ⬦ Child cuts out shapes. (See Appendix pp. 220-222 for shape cut outs.)
  ⬦ Child cuts out pictures.
+ Cutting textures: Child cuts out paper, cardboard, straw, playdough, and silly putty.
+ Child squeezes glue onto a line.

Handwriting Skills Involving Writing/Drawing

+ Child completes "dot-to-dots." (See Appendix pp. 237-241 for sample dot-to-dots.)
+ Child completes mazes. (See Appendix pp. 242-246 for varying level mazes.)
+ Child traces between lines or along shapes or pictures. (See Appendix pp. 247-251, 217-219, and 252-253 for tracing handouts.)
+ Handprint making: Child places nondominant hand on a piece of paper and uses the dominant hand to trace out the hand on the paper.
+ Child completes "follow the arrow" handout. (See Appendix p. 254 for sample handout.)
+ "Cage the animal": Therapist draws a picture of any animal inside a box. Therapist tells child that the animal will escape if bars are not drawn onto the animal's cage. Child draws straight lines from the top of the cage to the bottom of the cage.
+ Copying: Child copies different shapes, letters, words, sentences, or paragraphs onto a piece of paper.
+ Copying figures: Child copies a series of different complex figures and drawings. Keep in mind appropriate age expectations when having a child complete this activity. A child should not be asked to copy a figure that is developmentally too sophisticated. See the Beery Developmental Test of Visual Motor Integration as a resource for age appropriate expectations (Beery, Buktenica, & Beery, 2010).
+ Child uses stencils to make drawings and pictures.

Building

+ Child builds a house with Popsicle sticks (Figure 9-2).

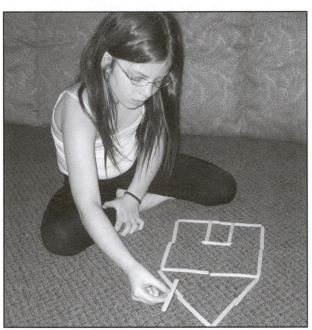

FIGURE 9-2

+ Create a box with Popsicle sticks: Therapist overlaps sticks on different layers and then has child copy the template design (Figure 9-3).

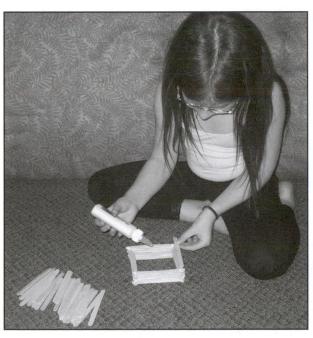

FIGURE 9-3

- Building/stacking: Child builds and stacks blocks and cubes to make a tower.
- Therapist creates a small design or tower with blocks or cubes and has child try to replicate the design or tower.
- Marshmallow building: Therapist creates different geometrical designs using marshmallows with toothpicks connecting the shape together. Child copies designs (Figure 9-4).

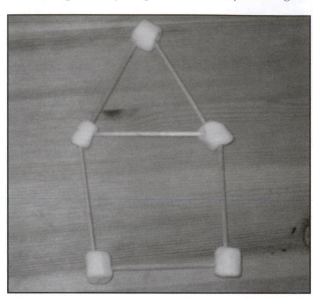

Figure 9-4

Forming Letters, Shapes, and Designs

- Pipe cleaner letters: Child copies models of letters with pipe cleaners and then creates letters independently with a pipe cleaner (without a model to look at).
- Playdough letters: Child copies letters with playdough and then creates letters independently with play-dough (without a model to look at).
- Therapist gives out Popsicle sticks. Child makes shapes and letters with Popsicle sticks.
- Child makes letters with Wikki Stix (Figure 9-5).

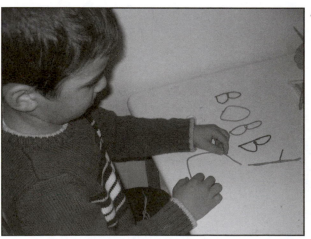

Figure 9-5

✦ Child copies designs and patterns with Wikki Stix (Figures 9-6 and 9-7). (See sample handout in Appendix p. 255 of designs child can copy with Wikki Stix.)

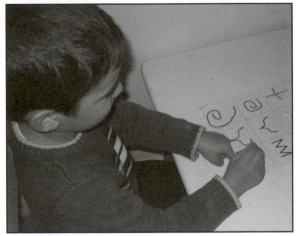

FIGURE 9-6

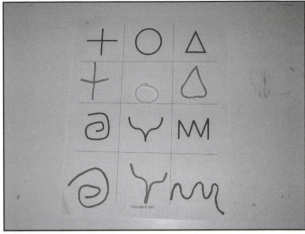

FIGURE 9-7

✦ Therapist cuts out different length pieces of string or colored lanyard and places the pieces overlapping in random patterns. Child tries to place strings in the same design as template (Figure 9-8).

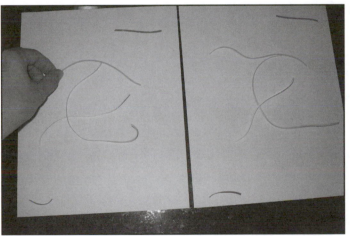

FIGURE 9-8

✦ Geoboards: Child copies designs and shapes on a Geoboard (Figure 9-9).

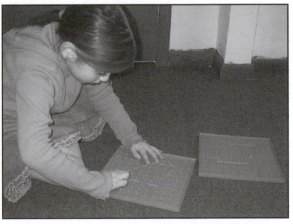

FIGURE 9-9

✦ Lacing boards: Child uses a lacing board and practices going around the lacing board with a whip stitch and then an over-under stitch.

◇ Whip stitch (Figure 9-10).

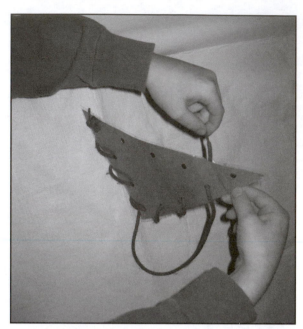

FIGURE 9-10

◇ Over-under stitch (Figure 9-11).

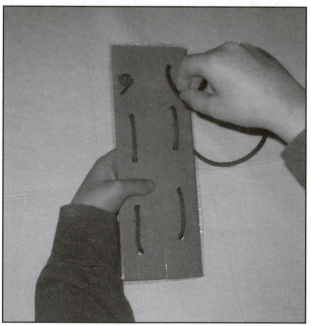

FIGURE 9-11

Ball Games

✦ Dribbling activities:
  ✧ Child practices dribbling a basketball quickly and slowly (Figure 9-12).

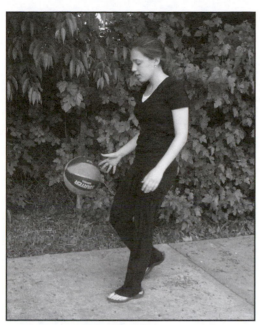

FIGURE 9-12

  ✧ Child practices dribbling a ball in each hand simultaneously (Figure 9-13).

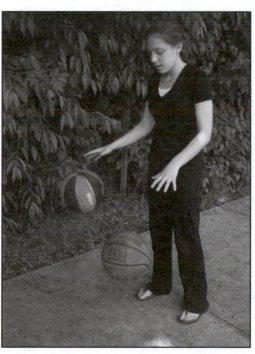

FIGURE 9-13

✦ HORSE: Child plays the basketball game HORSE with another child or therapist. Child shoots a ball in a basketball hoop. If the child misses the shot, it is the therapists turn. If the child makes the shot, the therapist must make the same shot. If the therapist misses, he/she gets a letter of the word "HORSE." If the therapist makes the shot, it is then the child's turn again to shoot a different shot, and so on. Whoever gets all letters and spells HORSE loses the game.

✦ Bowling: Therapist sets up bowling pins or soft blocks. Child uses a small- or medium-sized ball to bowl with and knocks over as many pins/blocks as possible.

✦ Juggling: Therapist teaches child how to juggle two or more balls (Figure 9-14).

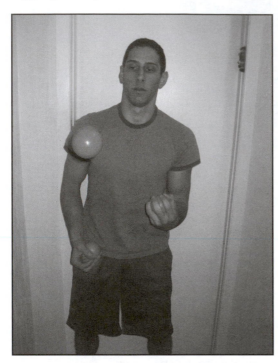

FIGURE 9-14

✦ Tic-Tock-Tire: Therapist hangs up a suspended tire swing (or a hula hoop) and swings it from side to side. Therapist places a bucket full of small items (bean bags, koosh balls, etc.) on the floor to the side of the child. Child picks up one item at a time and throws it through the moving tire without letting the bean bags touch the tire (Figure 9-15).

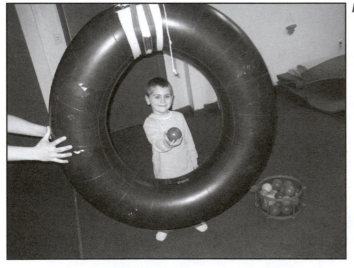

FIGURE 9-15

Folding Activities

✦ Origami: Therapist creates simple origami designs for child to copy.

✦ Paper airplanes: Therapist creates a paper airplane and has child copy the steps, one step at a time.

✦ Dinner napkin folding: Therapist teaches child simple ways to fold dinner napkins. Different fun ideas can be found on the Web by searching for "easy napkin folding."

On the Web

✦ Visit www.eyecanlearn.com for additional visual motor activities that can be played on a computer.

COMMERCIALLY AVAILABLE PRODUCTS

✦ "Jacks"

✦ "Labyrinth Game"

✦ "Frisbee"

✦ "Elefun"

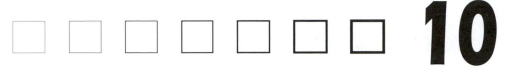

Visual Scanning

Visual scanning is the ability of the eyes to work together to track a moving or stationary target. Although visual scanning refers to a set of skills that encompasses many different areas, this section will focus on a few specific components of visual scanning. These specific components include tracking a slow-moving object, moving the eyes quickly between two different close objects, and moving the eyes from an object that is close to an object that is far back.

Poor visual scanning will result in many academic and functional deficits. Academically, reading and sentence copying will be most affected. Functionally, a child will have difficulty playing sports and simply being able to watch moving objects in the environment.

Children with poor visual scanning skills will often compensate for this deficit by moving the head instead of using isolated eye movements when tracking something. This results in inefficient and ineffective visual scanning. When performing the activities in this chapter, it is important to remind the children to keep the head still. It may also be necessary to provide gentle physical input to serve as a reminder to keep the head still during some exercises. If the head moves when these exercises are performed, then the children will not be improving visual scanning abilities to the optimal level.

In this chapter, multiple visual scanning exercises are provided. Included is a group of exercises that involves visual scanning activities involving balance. The reason these exercises are incorporated into this chapter is that a child's environment is a constantly moving one. Children must learn to visually scan on static surfaces as well as dynamic ones. For example, a child might want to read a street sign while walking on a bumpy sidewalk, ascending a flight of stairs, or stepping up onto a curb.

It is also important to know that the visual system has a strong connection to the system in one's body that controls movement. When performing visual scanning exercises a therapist must watch for signs of dizziness and stop immediately if a child reports being either dizzy or nauseous.

Danto, A., & Pruzansky, M. *1001 Pediatric Treatment Activities: Creative Ideas for Therapy Sessions* (pp. 83-90).
© 2011 SLACK Incorporated

Visual Scanning Activities

Basic Visual Tracking

✦ Visual tracking for higher-level child: Therapist holds an object in front of child's face. Therapist instructs child to look at the moving object with only the eyes and not to move the head. Therapist should alternate moving the object slowly and quickly in all different planes. (Try to pick something visually attractive in order to help the child maintain visual attention.)

✦ Visual tracking for lower-level child or young child (to be determined by therapist): Place child in upright, seated position or flat on back. Move a toy/object of interest/shining light around child. Move the toy or light in an arc from side to side, up and down, and in both diagonal planes.

    ✧ On back: (Figures 10-1 through 10-3).

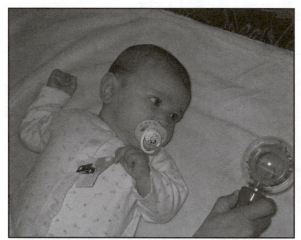

FIGURE 10-1

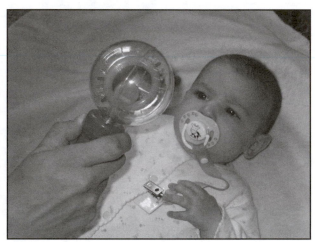

FIGURE 10-2

FIGURE 10-3

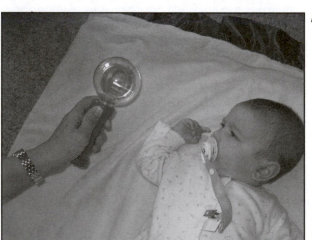

✧ Sitting upright: (Figures 10-4 through 10-6).

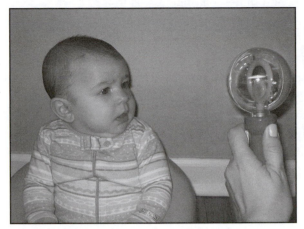

FIGURE 10-4

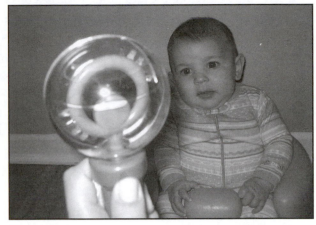

FIGURE 10-5

FIGURE 10-6

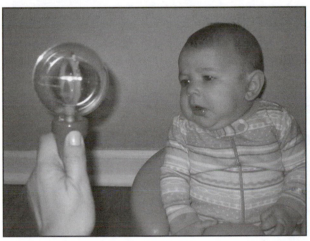

✦ Practicing saccades (i.e., the ability to quickly move the eyes from one target to another): Therapist holds up one object in each hand and has child alternate looking at each object in a random pattern. For example, therapist can hold a red marble and a blue marble. Therapist then calls out "red, blue, red, blue, etc." Therapist moves the two objects around/up/down while child looks back and forth between them, while keeping the head still (Figure 10-7).

FIGURE 10-7

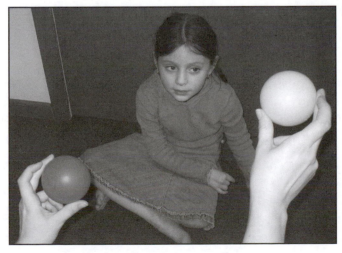

◆ Flashlight Tag: This game should be played in a dark room. Therapist shines a light on the ceiling or somewhere else in the room. Child quickly locates this light and shines a flashlight next to it.

> *Note: In order to increase isolated eye movements instead of full head movements, it might be helpful to lightly hold child's head still, forcing child to only move the eyes and not the head.*

◆ "Where is it": Therapist places a penny or small object on the table in front of child. Therapist picks it up with one hand and transfers it back and forth between hands several times as the child watches. When the therapist stops, child must guess which hand is holding the penny.

◆ Reading exercises:

◇ Child holds book in hand and reads out loud to therapist.

◇ Child reads book keeping the index finger under the word being read.

◇ Child reads a row of letters placed on the board X feet away. (Appropriate distance should be determined by treating therapist.)

◇ Child reads a list of sentences placed on the wall X feet away. (Appropriate distance should be determined by treating therapist.)

◆ "Where is the queen": Therapist places three playing cards face up on the table. One of the cards should be a queen. Therapist shows the child where the queen is and then turns the cards face down. Therapist slowly moves the cards around and then the child has to point to the card that he/she believes the queen is under.

◆ Bead mazes: Child completes bead maze (Figure 10-8).

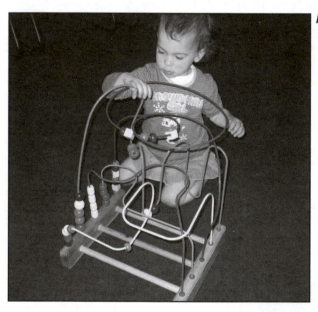

Figure 10-8

Visual Scanning Activities Involving Balance

◆ Balance beam scanning game: Child walks across a balance beam while reading across a row on a letter chart placed on the wall at the child's front or side. To upgrade this activity, have child read down a column, read the first and last letters of a row, read every other letter in a row, or read two letters at a time. This activity can be made simpler by placing a long strip of masking tape on the floor and having the child walk across the masking tape instead of the balance beam when reading the letters. If a child does not yet know the names of the letters, an alternative picture/symbol chart can be used. (See Appendix pp. 256-257 for letter and symbol chart.)

◆ Slow movement tips: Child sits in a chair facing therapist. Therapist holds child's head and maintains eye contact with child. Therapist slowly moves child's head in different directions, including right, left, backward, and forward.

✦ Heel-toe rocking: Child maintains balance on heels. Child then rocks back and forth between heels and toes, holding each position for approximately one to two seconds. Once child is able to perform this activity smoothly, therapist places a sentence on the wall that child must read while rocking back and forth between heels and toes.

Writing/Drawing

✦ Matching cars games: Therapist takes a piece of paper and on the far right side of the page makes a column with different cars and on the far left side of the page writes different numbers. Draw lines between the cars and numbers and ask the child to use only his/her eyes to see where each vehicle ended up. (See Appendix pp. 258-260 for sample handouts.)

✦ Copying words and sentences: Child copies words or sentences from a blackboard onto a paper placed on a table or desk in front of the child.

✦ Copying words and sentences: Child copies words or sentences out of a book placed on the table directly in front of the child.

✦ Blowing bubbles: Child stands on floor or on a balance beam. Therapist blows bubbles all around child. Child tries to pop as many bubbles as possible.

Throw/Catch and Ball Activities

✦ Child throws a hula hoop in the air and catches it (Figure 10-9).

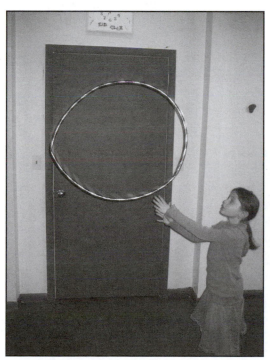

FIGURE 10-9

✦ Hula hoop toss: Child and therapist both hold a hula hoop in their hands. When therapist calls out "go," they each throw their hula hoop and catch the other person's hula hoop simultaneously (Figure 10-10).

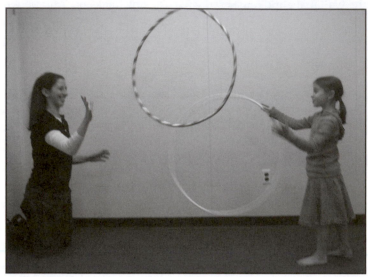

FIGURE 10-10

✦ ABC wall game: Therapist places the letters A through E on the wall approximately half an inch apart in a random order. The letters should be large enough so a child can stand a few feet away from the wall and still see them. Child throws a ball at letter "A" and catches it. Then continues throwing it at the next letter and catches it. Therapist can upgrade this activity by adding more letters or downgrade the activity by only placing two or three letters on the wall.

✦ Wall spelling game: Therapist places scattered letters on the wall in a random order. Therapist calls out a letter and child throws a ball against the corresponding letter and catches it. For older children, therapist calls out a word and child throws the ball at each letter in the word (in the correct order).

✦ Child plays a sports game that requires a quick moving ball. Some of these activities include floor hockey, air hockey, miniature golf, ping pong, Frisbee, soccer, hitting a baseball in the air, tennis, etc. (Figure 10-11).

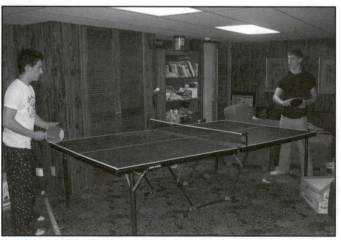

FIGURE 10-11

✦ Balloon air-bouncing: Child hits a balloon with either a racquet or own hand. Child tries to keep the balloon from falling to the floor.

✦ Balloon volleyball: Child hits a balloon with either a racquet or own hand while playing a game of volleyball with another person.

✦ Child bounces a small ball between a tennis racket and the floor.

✦ Child bounces a small ball on top of a tennis racket and keeps it in the air.

Jumping

+ Trampoline letter game: Therapist tapes different letters onto a trampoline. Therapist calls out one letter at a time and child quickly finds the letter and jumps onto it.
+ Arrow map: Therapist places arrow map on the wall. (See Appendix p. 261 for sample chart.) Child reads the directions of the arrows out loud, walks in the direction of the arrows, jumps in the direction the arrows, or dances to a beat while moving in the direction of the arrows.

Strengthening Eye Convergence

+ Therapist places a small sticker on the wall. Child does wall push-ups while maintaining eye contact on the sticker and has nose touch the sticker each time the body is brought in close to the wall (Figure 10-12).

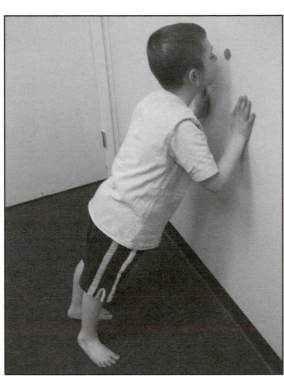

FIGURE 10-12

✦ Suspended ball activities: Child hits a suspended ball or tether ball with hand or any sort of rod. Upgrade the activity by taping colored lines on a rod and have child only hit the ball with a specific color. Further upgrade this activity by performing it on a balance board (Figure 10-13).

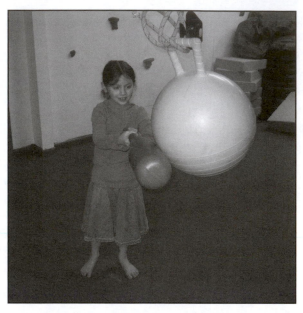

FIGURE 10-13

✦ Child throws a small ball high up in the air and catches it. Upgrade this activity by performing it on a balance board.

✦ Child throws a ball against the wall and catches it without letting the ball drop on floor.

✦ Swing basketball: Therapist places a small basketball hoop next to a platform swing and places small bean bags or Koosh balls around the perimeter of the swing. Child stands on the swing and picks up one piece at a time to throw into the basketball hoop. Therapist slowly swings the child back and forth; the child faces the direction of the basketball hoop while playing this game.

On the Web

✦ Visit www.eyecanlearn.com for additional visual scanning exercises.

✦ Visit http://abcteach.com and follow links for mazes and Dot-to-Dot handouts.

COMMERCIALLY AVAILABLE PRODUCTS

✦ "Lucky Ducks"

✦ "Zoom Ball"

✦ "Simon"

DISSOCIATION ACTIVITIES

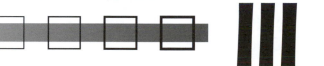

III

Dissociation refers to the ability to use individual parts of the body in isolation from the rest of the body. When a child has decreased dissociation, movements will appear stiff and clumsy. There are different forms of dissociation. In the upcoming chapters of this section, body dissociation and finger individuation will be discussed.

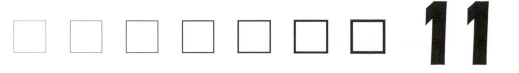

BODY DISSOCIATION

Body dissociation refers to the ability to move one part of the body without moving another part. For example, when a child rolls over, the child should be able to segmentally roll his/her body by dissociating the right and left extremities as well as dissociating the extremities and the head. A child with poor body dissociation will move stiffly—like a log—in one unit, as opposed to a segmental roll (Tecklin, 2008).

Poor body dissociation will result in stiff and uncoordinated movement. This will also cause a child to use inefficient movement patterns. Inefficient movement patterns require more energy expenditure on the child's part and take an increased amount of time. When children are playing and moving within their environments, movement should be quick, simple, and not require a large amount of energy.

There are three main components to body dissociation: the ability to move parts of the upper body and lower body separately, the ability to move an extremity in isolation from the body and from the other extremity, and the ability to move the head and facial muscles in isolation from each other. This chapter will provide activities to improve the three different components of body dissociation.

This chapter also discusses exercises to work on torticollis—a condition commonly associated with small children that involves tight neck muscles. The reason these exercises are provided in this chapter is that a child with tight neck muscles will have difficulty dissociating his/her head and neck from the rest of the body and may subsequently present with overall difficulties with general dissociation.

Danto, A., & Pruzansky, M. *1001 Pediatric Treatment Activities:*
Creative Ideas for Therapy Sessions (pp. 93-98).
© 2011 SLACK Incorporated

Body Dissociation Treatment Activities

Whole Body Dissociation

✦ Baseball: Therapist places a baseball or Wiffle ball on a tee. Child practices swinging a bat. While this game can also be played without a tee, it will be easier to work on dissociating the different trunk muscles if the ball is hit off the tee in a slow and controlled fashion (as opposed to swinging at a ball in the air).

✦ Place child (developmentally 6-14 months) (Cottrell, 2004, p. 19) on side and place a toy in front of child in order to motivate child to fully roll over (Figure 11-1).

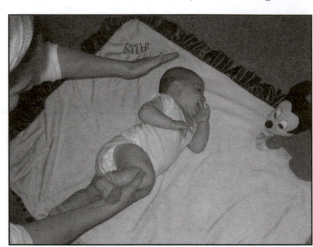

FIGURE 11-1

✦ Twist child's legs toward desired side to be rolled in order to give child a head start (Figure 11-2).

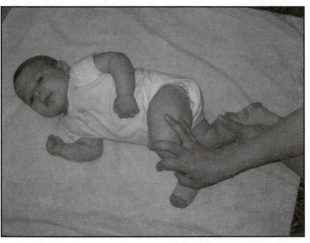

FIGURE 11-2

✦ Rolling: Child slowly rolls on a mat segmentally (first head, then trunk, then legs), not like a log. If child appears stiff while rolling, therapist can provide child with verbal and physical cuing as needed.

✦ Fast running: Child runs across the room or outside. Therapist can remind child to utilize an arm swing when running.

✦ Frog jump activities: Child squats down on the floor and frog jumps as far as possible. Child jumps to a basket and places Koosh balls or other toys in it to make this activity more playful.

Dissociating Extremities From the Body

◆ Dry-wet game: Therapist wets different parts of child's body with water, alternating between wetting a part on the child's right side and left side (e.g., arms, fingers, shoulders, knees, etc.). Therapist calls out a body part that is wet ("wet hand") and child must extend/raise only the body part that is wet while keeping the dry counter body part down.

◆ Child moves both arms three to four times in a specific direction (in and out, up and down, to the side, etc.). Therapist then asks child to only move one side in that same direction and motion. This game can also be played with the lower extremities.

  ◇ Position 1 (Figure 11-3), Position 2 (Figure 11-4), Position 3 (Figure 11-5).

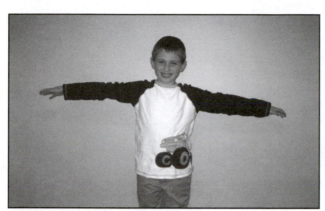

FIGURE 11-3

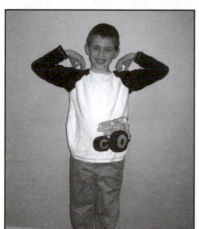

FIGURE 11-4

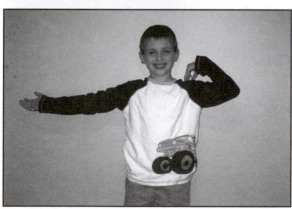

FIGURE 11-5

- ✦ Child lays on the floor or stands against the wall. Child lifts one leg or arm at a time off the floor or wall, while keeping the other limb flush against the resting surface.
- ✦ Child stands still with both hands on hips and kicks a moving ball.
- ✦ Child shrugs one shoulder at a time.
- ✦ Child lies on floor or outdoors in snow and makes snow angels. Child then attempts to do this, but only on one side at a time.
- ✦ Child turns a jump rope with one hand (therapist can tie a rope to a doorknob or hold the other end of the rope), while keeping the rest of the body still (Figure 11-6).

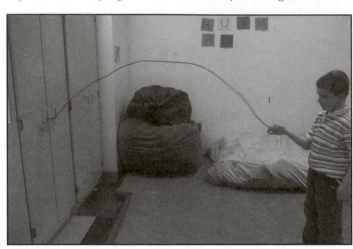

FIGURE 11-6

- ✦ Coloring activity: In order to help a child use isolated wrist/finger movements instead of whole arm movements when coloring a large picture, therapist can divide a picture into many smaller sections. If the child is able to follow instructions and only color in one section at a time, this will automatically cause the child to use more isolated movements when coloring (Figure 11-7).

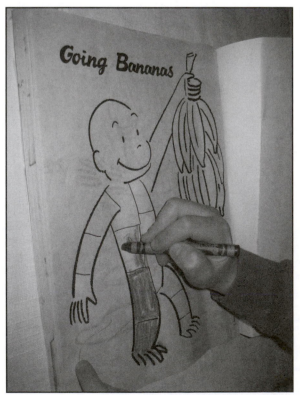

FIGURE 11-7

Dissociating Head and Facial Muscles

- ✦ Child visually tracks a moving target while keeping the head still.
- ✦ Child shakes head "yes" and "no" without moving the shoulders or any part of the trunk.
- ✦ Child moves head all around in a circle, keeping the rest of the body still.
- ✦ Child moves one side of the facial muscles at a time to wink, close an eye, blow up one cheek, or move the lips. Child then switches and makes the same movements using only the muscles on the other side of the face (Figures 11-8 and 11-9).

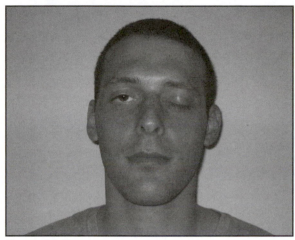

FIGURE 11-8

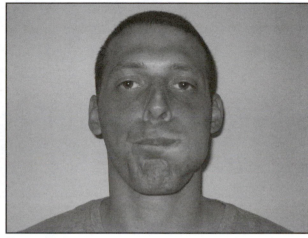

FIGURE 11-9

Treating Torticollis

- ✦ Massage child's tight neck muscles with lotion.
- ✦ Elongate and stretch child's tight neck muscles (Figures 11-10 and 11-11).

   *Do not perform any stretches on child without first being taught how to properly handle and stretch child by either a doctor or a trained occupational or physical therapist. Repeat at each diaper change.

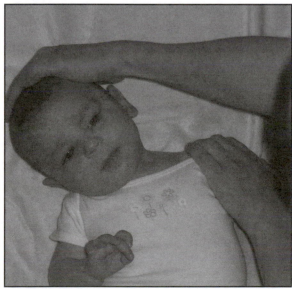

FIGURE 11-10

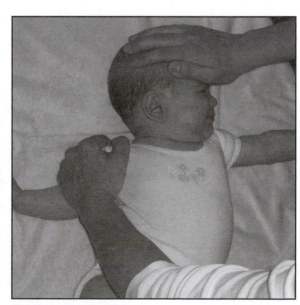

FIGURE 11-11

✦ Have child face the nonpreferred side: Stimulate nonpreferred by either placing a toy for child to look at or having an adult play peek-a-boo on nonpreferred side. Child can be sitting, lying on back, belly, or on your lap on child's belly (Figure 11-12).

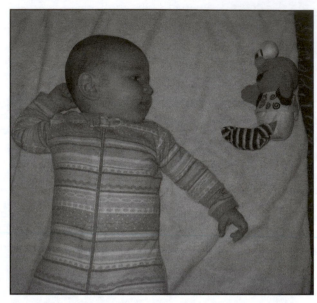

FIGURE 11-12

✦ Place stroller toys toward the nonpreferred side of the child during walks.

✦ When child is sleeping, turn child's head to nonpreferred side.

✦ Have child play in side-lying position.

✦ Increase tummy time. See Chapter 19, Upper Arm Strengthening and Stabilization, for a list of ways to help increase child's tolerance toward tummy time.

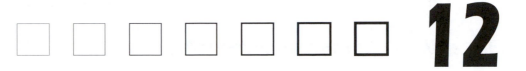

FINGER INDIVIDUATION

Finger individuation is the ability to move a single finger in isolation from the other fingers. Finger individuation is needed for many everyday activities, such as holding a writing utensil, typing, grasping a key to turn a lock, self-care, and engaging in most fine motor activities. Accurately coordinating finger movements is also necessary in order to approximate the size, shape, and use of an object before making contact with a particular object (Raghavan, Krakauer, Santello & Gordon, 2007). Some children are unable to move an individual finger in isolation from the other fingers on the hand and, therefore, cannot master a needed level of precision during fine motor activities.

This chapter provides activities that require isolated finger use and will promote improved hand and finger function.

Danto, A., & Pruzansky, M. *1001 Pediatric Treatment Activities:*
Creative Ideas for Therapy Sessions (pp. 99-104).
© 2011 SLACK Incorporated

Finger Individuation Treatment Activities

Playful Finger Games

✦ Child sings "Where is Thumpkin?" while holding up the appropriate finger:

> Where is Thumpkin, where is thumpkin?
> *Chorus:*
> Here I am, here I am.
> How are you today sir?
> Very well I thank you.
> Run away, run away.

◇ Follow with "pointer," "tall man," "ring man," and "pinky."

✦ Therapist and child play "This Little Piggy…": Child sticks out one finger at a time for therapist when playing this game (Figure 12-1).

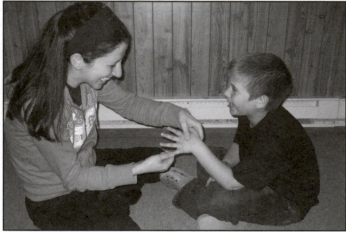

Figure 12-1

✦ Counting: Child counts out loud with fingers, one number at a time. Child counts forward to 10 and then backward.

✦ Therapist places finger puppets on child's fingers. Child then acts out a story.

✦ Thumb wars.

> *This game should only be played between therapist and child, not between two children, in order to ensure no one gets hurt.*

Computer and Keyboard Activities

✦ Child plays computer games that involve pushing specific buttons with specific fingers.

✦ Child plays computer games that require use of a mouse: Many children have difficulty using a mouse because they are unable to push down with their index fingers in isolation, and instead push down with both fingers together.

✦ Typing: Child writes words and sentences or a story with the keyboard keys.

✦ Child plays a song on a piano or keyboard. If this is too challenging, child can copy/imitate hitting specifics notes on the piano.

Crafts and Coloring

+ Finger crayons:
  ◇ Therapist places a different finger crayon on each of child's fingers. Child colors a picture with finger crayons.
  ◇ Therapist places finger crayons on each of child's fingers. Therapist tells child to make a line, but only with a specific color. Therapist then asks child to make a line, by choosing two colors that should be used together at the same time.
+ Child peels stickers off of a sticker sheet and places them on a piece of paper.
+ Child colors in or traces gradually smaller shapes.
+ Bead games: Therapist places a small bead between the child's index finger and thumb. Child rolls the bead back and forth and side to side. Child then transfers bead between the next finger and thumb and performs the same activity. Child continues to the pinky and then works back towards the thumb.
+ Playdough/Theraputty: Child pushes one finger at a time down into the putty.
+ Child strings beads to make a necklace.
+ Child crumples small pieces of tissue paper with one hand, using only the finger tips to crumple the paper.
+ Child writes letters in small graph paper boxes (Figures 12-2 and 12-3).

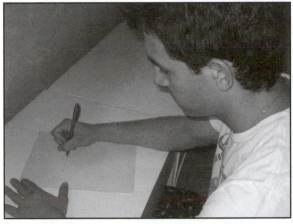

FIGURE 12-2

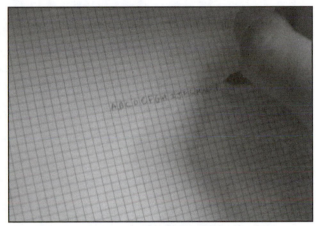

FIGURE 12-3

Finger Exercises and Positions

+ Child touches each finger to the thumb one at a time (Figure 12-4).

FIGURE 12-4

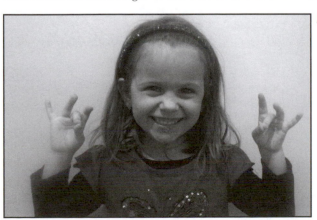

◆ Child imitates different hand and finger positions.

◆ Finger writing: Child pretends that his/her fingertip is a pencil and writes a word on a piece of paper using only the fingertip. Therapist may need to gently stabilize child's hand so that only the finger and the finger-tips move to write the letters. (This activity may be difficult for some children and a child may resist using fine finger movements. The supervising therapist should only use gentle guidance when assisting any child in this activity.)

◆ Child carries multiple items in each hand. Child uses the fingers to wrap around each item (around a loop, bag strap, hula hoop, pen, or anything that can be gripped with just the fingers). Therapist calls out one item and child must release that item without dropping other items in the hand (Figures 12-5 and 12-6). An alternative way to play this game is with paper. Child holds different colored strips of construction paper between each finger. Therapist calls out a color and child must drop the specific color without releasing any other color.

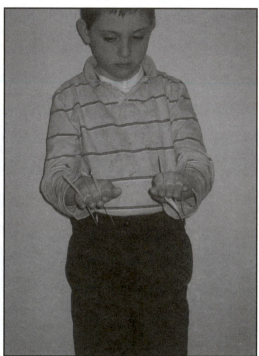

FIGURE 12-5

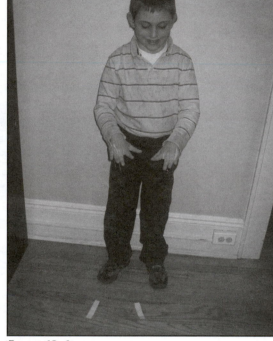

FIGURE 12-6

Using the Thumb and Index Finger Together

◆ Child picks up small pellet sized objects.

◆ Page turning: Child turns the pages of a story book, one page at a time.

◆ Card dealing: Child deals out a deck of cards using only one hand at a time, thereby forcing the child to isolate thumb movements when dealing out the cards.

◆ Child twirls a pen around the fingers.

◆ Spin a top: Child practices spinning a top on a tabletop, floor, or other hard surface.

Playing Musical Instruments

✦ Therapist teaches child some notes or chords on any instrument with strings including:
  ✧ Guitar, violin, cello, etc. (Figure 12-7).

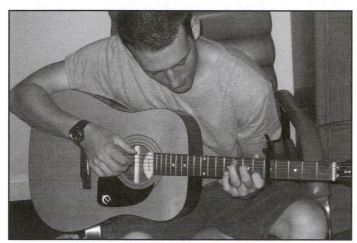

FIGURE 12-7

✦ Therapist teaches child some notes or chords on any instrument with buttons or holes to press or cover, including:
  ✧ Recorder, horn instruments, brass instruments.

COMMERCIALLY AVAILABLE PRODUCTS

✦ "Etch-a-Sketch"

HAND SKILLS

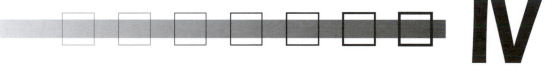

IV

Hand skills are important skills needed for everyday functioning with gross motor tasks as well as tasks involving fine precision. This section includes activities that will assist in improving functional hand use by focusing on the necessary prerequisites needed for this skill. This section will also focus on placing the hand and fingers in the correct position when engaged in a fine motor activity and playing games with very small objects that require precision. Finally, it will focus on strengthening the small muscles of the hand, as well as practicing skills that involve those muscles, such as grasping a sock to pull it on, coloring with a crayon, or engaging in craft activities.

OPEN WEBSPACE

An open webspace (Figure 13-1) is the space created between the thumb and the index finger when the index finger is in a proper position of opposition with the thumb when grasping an object. A closed webspace usually indicates that a child has decreased thumb stability. When children have decreased thumb or finger stability, they will often compensate for this in two different ways. One way will result in a child grasping a pencil with an awkward pencil grasp, causing poor handwriting. The other way is that children will try to stabilize their hands by using too much force and energy when writing. This will cause the child to fatigue quickly and the work product will suffer.

This chapter will provide two different types of activities. First, there are activities that promote moving the different fingers to the tip of the thumb, promoting opposition, thereby opening the webspace. The second type of activity involves wrapping the child's hands around different objects, naturally creating an open webspace. The activities provided in this chapter are intended to help a child promote the finger and hand stability needed for precision and fine motor skills.

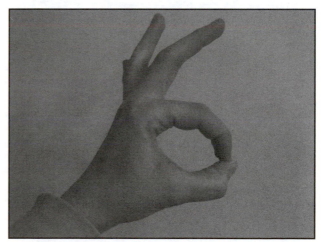

FIGURE 13-1

Danto, A., & Pruzansky, M. *1001 Pediatric Treatment Activities: Creative Ideas for Therapy Sessions* (pp. 107-110).
© 2011 SLACK Incorporated

Activities To Open Webspace

Exercises

+ Child touches each finger to the thumb, going forward, backward, and then on both hands simultaneously.
+ Making "Oh's": Child practices forming the letter "O" with the webspace.
+ Stretching exercises: Therapist gently massages and then stretches the webspace open for the child.
+ "Finger Twister": Therapist creates mini Twister board and has child play twister with the fingers.

Special Equipment

+ Child uses different pencil grippers when writing or coloring in order to help keep the webspace open during activities with a writing utensil.

Wrapping the Hands Around Round Objects

+ Wrap hand around:
  ◇ Small balls (Figure 13-2).

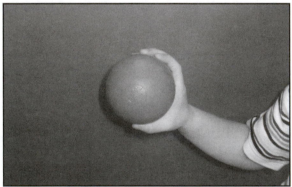

FIGURE 13-2

  ◇ Handles on a bike (Figure 13-3).

FIGURE 13-3

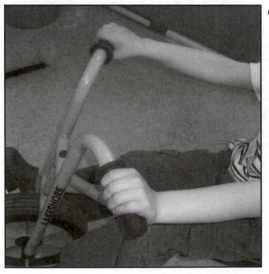

- ❖ Rungs on a ladder in the playground.
- ❖ Rungs on the monkey bars in a playground (Figure 13-4).

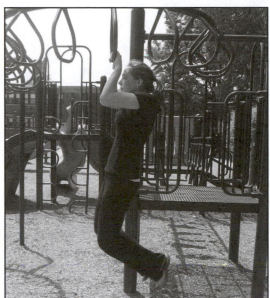

FIGURE 13-4

- ❖ Around trampoline handle bars (Figure 13-5).

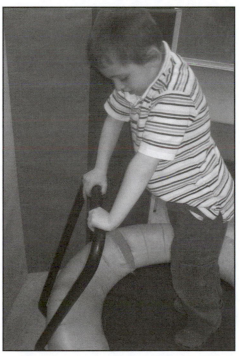

FIGURE 13-5

✧ Around jump rope handles (Figure 13-6).

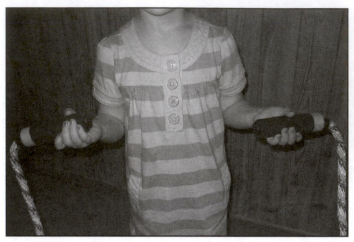

FIGURE 13-6

✦ Use a roller to flatten dough.
✦ Hold onto ropes while on platform swing.
✦ Hold onto trapeze bar (Figure 13-7).

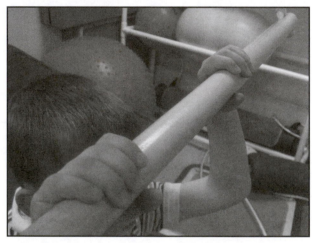

FIGURE 13-7

✦ Sit on seesaw and hold onto handle bars.
✦ Child holds pencil with proper grasp, while therapist encourages an open webspace (Figure 13-8).

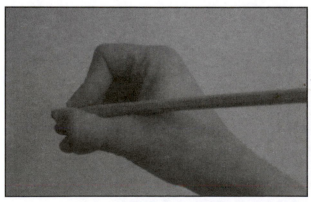

FIGURE 13-8

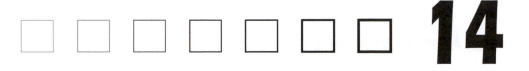

FINE MOTOR

Fine motor skills are skills that involve a refined use of the small muscles controlling the hand, fingers, and thumb. The development of these skills allows one to be able to complete such tasks as writing, drawing, picking up small objects, and buttoning one's shirt.

The following chapter provides activities that will assist in strengthening fine motor skills by engaging a child in games and activities with small parts and pieces. The purpose of the suggested activities is to improve overall dexterity of the hands. The activities provided require a child to use in-hand manipulation, pincer grasp, and other finger manipulative skills.

Danto, A., & Pruzansky, M. *1001 Pediatric Treatment Activities:*
Creative Ideas for Therapy Sessions (pp. 111-118).
© 2011 SLACK Incorporated

Fine Motor Activities

Theraputty/Playdough

◆ Child makes little balls out of Theraputty or playdough by rolling small pieces between the fingertips. Child then picks up pieces with tongs and places them into a nearby container.

◆ Child finds the letters of own name on letter beads. Child then hides those specific letter beads in Theraputty or playdough and subsequently finds them.

Writing/Coloring

◆ Finger crayons: Child colors and makes a picture with finger crayons placed on specific fingers (Figures 14-1 and 14-2).

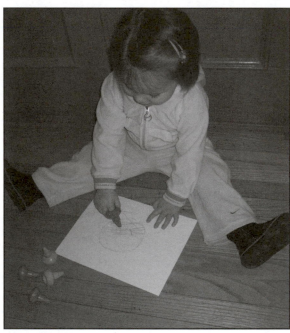

Figure 14-1

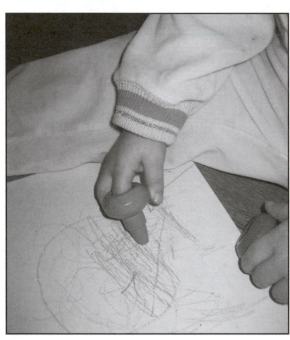

Figure 14-2

✦ Toothpicks activity: Therapist traces child's name lightly on a piece of Styrofoam board with a pencil or pen. Child places toothpicks, one at a time, into Styrofoam along the traced letters of name to poke holes (Figure 14-3). Child then colors over the letters (Figure 14-4).

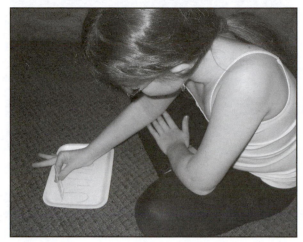

FIGURE 14-3

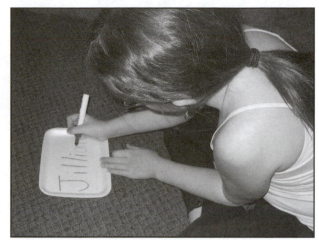

FIGURE 14-4

Beading and Lacing Activities

✦ Pop beads:
  ✧ Child pushes and connects small pop beads together. Child then pulls beads apart one at a time (Figures 14-5 and 14-6).

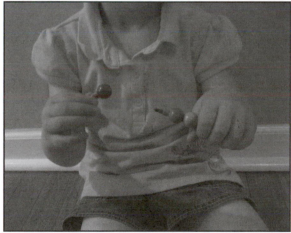

FIGURE 14-5

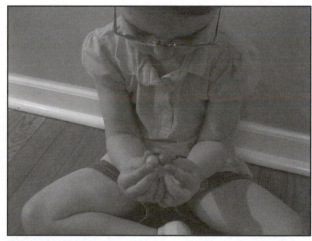

FIGURE 14-6

✧ Child pushes and connects large pop beads together. Child then pulls beads apart one at a time (Figures 14-7 and 14-8).

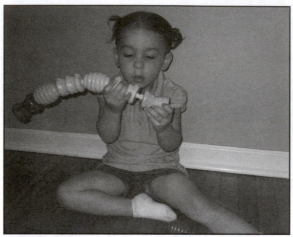 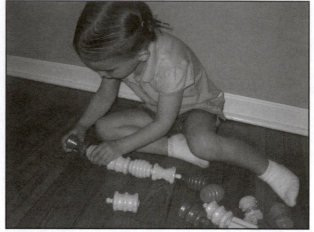

FIGURE 14-7 *FIGURE 14-8*

+ Food art: Child strings macaroni to make a necklace, bracelet, or another design.
+ Froot Loops necklace: Child strings Froot Loops on a long, thin piece of licorice. (This activity can also be played with Cheerios.)
+ Lacing beads: Child strings beads on a thin piece of string. (If this is too challenging, this activity can be downgraded by stringing the beads onto a pipe cleaner.)
+ Bead rolling: Therapist places a small bead between child's index finger and thumb. Child rolls the bead back and forth, side to side, and then in circles. Child then tries to transfer bead between the next finger and thumb and perform the same activity. Child continues to the pinky and works back toward the thumb.
+ Lacing art and sewing kits: Therapist teaches child different sewing stitches (whip stitch/over-under stitch) with a needle and thread. (Make sure the needle is not too sharp and that this activity is only performed with a child with appropriate safety awareness.)

Peeling With the Fingertips

+ Child peels strips of masking tape off of a tape roll. Child makes shapes, letters, or a picture with the different strips of paper. (This activity is often more fun for a child when colored masking tape is used.)
+ Child peels stickers off of a sticker sheet and places them on a piece of paper.
+ Button Candy: Therapist gives child a reward with Button Candy and has child peel the candy off the sheet of paper (Figure 14-9).

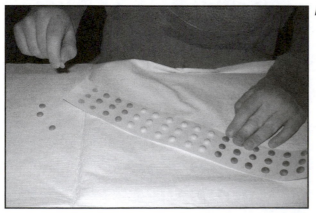

FIGURE 14-9

+ Turning pages: Therapist reads child a book. Child turns the pages with fingertips.
+ Pop-up books: Therapist reads child a pop-up book. Child lifts tabs off the page with finger tips.
+ Child peels an orange or grapefruit and then may eat it.
+ Cookie cutters: Child pushes cookie-cutter into dough and then peels out cookie shape by pulling away excess dough.

Manipulating Small Objects

+ Grasp release activities (developmental age 7 to 9 months):
  ◇ Therapist places toy fish in a small toy fishbowl and has child take each fish out of fishbowl and then put them back in one at a time. (The Ocean Wonders Musical Fishbowl plays music to reinforce putting in and taking out the fish, which may make this activity more reinforcing to the child.)
  ◇ Therapist takes a simple bucket and several toys that the child enjoys playing with. Therapist places toys in the bucket. The child removes the toys one at a time and then places them back in the bucket. Repeat several times.
+ Child attaches paper clips in a chain.
+ Nuts and bolts: Child screws together different sized nuts and bolts.
+ Therapist scatters several pennies/coins on table. Child picks up three coins, one at a time. Child places each coin, one at a time, back into a piggy bank. (In order to upgrade this activity to work on in-hand manipulation and translation, increase the number of pennies the child must pick up at one time).
+ Penny flipping: Therapist places ten pennies on the table in a line. Child turns each penny over, one at a time.
+ Penny design making: Child creates different pictures and designs using pennies.
+ Penny picture handouts: Child picks up one penny at a time and places the pennies onto the circular marks on the Penny Flipping Handout to make a design. (See Appendix pp. 262-264 for sample penny handouts).

Cutting Activities

+ Therapist draws lines, shapes, or animals onto a piece of paper. Child practices cutting along the lines in order to cut out the picture. If this is too challenging, therapist can hold a 1-inch strip of paper and allow child to make snips in the paper. (See Appendix pages 217-222 for sample cutting activity pages.)

Keys

+ Lock and key: Therapist provides child with different keys. Child unlocks different doors or locked boxes.
+ Child adds keys onto a key chain ring. (The larger the key chain ring, the easier the activity.)

Games

+ Therapist demonstrates "cause and effect" toy where the child has to press/pull/push a knob or button in order to make a character pop up (developmental age 6 to 9 months).

✦ Dominoes: Child creates a long line of dominoes on a flat surface and then tips the last domino to watch the domino effect. It may be necessary to assist child in this task in order to make sure the child does not accidentally knock a domino over too early (Figures 14-10 through 14-12).

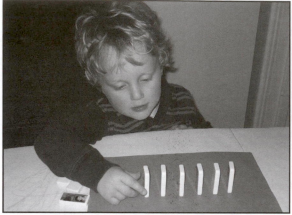

FIGURE 14-10

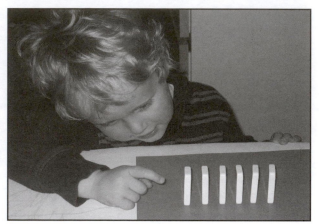

FIGURE 14-11

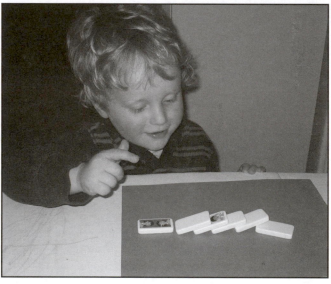

FIGURE 14-12

✦ Card flipping: Therapist plays a card game or a game of memory in which child must flip cards over on the table. (Do not let the child drag the card to the edge of the table in order to flip it over or else child will not be using the small muscles in the fingers for the card-flipping task.)

✦ Travel-sized games: Child plays travel-sized games with small pieces. Some examples include:

    ◇ Checkers.

    ◇ Chess.

    ◇ Connect Four.

Dressing and Grooming

- ✦ Doll dressing: Child plays with small dolls in order to dress and undress them.
- ✦ Dressing skills and manipulating fasteners. Child can engage in:
  - ✧ Tying and untying shoe laces.
  - ✧ Buttoning and unbuttoning shirt.
  - ✧ Buckling and unbuckling belt buckles.
  - ✧ Zipping and unzipping zippers.
  - ✧ Snapping and unsnapping snaps.
  - ✧ Hooking overall latches and unhooking.
- ✦ "Don't drop the clothes": Therapist places multiple skirts or pants on skirt hanger. Child tries to hold hanger up in the air and remove one article of clothing from the skirt hanger without letting the other articles of clothing fall on the floor (Figure 14-13).

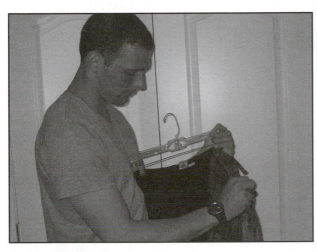

FIGURE 14-13

- ✦ Folding activities: therapist teaches child how to fold clothing neatly into a pile (Figure 14-14).

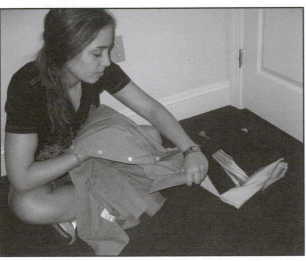

FIGURE 14-14

◆ Makeup application: Therapist teaches older girls how to apply makeup.
◆ Nail polish: Therapist and child practice polishing fingers or toes (Figure 14-15).

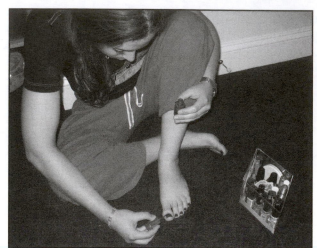

FIGURE 14-15

COMMERCIALLY AVAILABLE PRODUCTS

◆ "Mastermind"
◆ "Lite Brite"
◆ "Mancala"
◆ "ADL books"
◆ "Melissa & Doug" Latches Puzzle
◆ "Melissa & Doug" Basic Skills Board
◆ "Bead art"
◆ "Cheerios Book"
◆ "Tinkertoys"
◆ "Hi-Ho Cherry-O"
◆ "Cootie Game"
◆ "Don't Spill the Beans"
◆ "Perler Beads"

PINCH GRASP MANIPULATION

15

Pinch grasp manipulation is the ability to pinch an object between the tip of the thumb and the pointer finger and then manipulate the object in any way needed. This would be required when picking up small, pellet-sized items such as raisins, holding onto the laces when tying a shoe, or putting coins into a piggy bank. Many children have the fine motor skills needed to use a pincer grasp, but lack the necessary strength. The following chapter will discuss ways to work on strengthening the pinch grasp (pincer grasp).

Danto, A., & Pruzansky, M. *1001 Pediatric Treatment Activities: Creative Ideas for Therapy Sessions* (pp. 119-124).
© 2011 SLACK Incorporated

Pinch Grasp Manipulation

Pincer Activities

✦ Child colors with small broken pieces of crayons (Figure 15-1). This automatically places child's fingers in correct pincer position for coloring and prewriting activities.

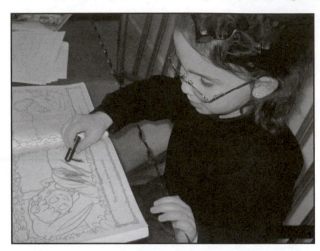

FIGURE 15-1

✦ Child colors with adapted pencil grips and graspers placed on writing utensil (Figure 15-2).

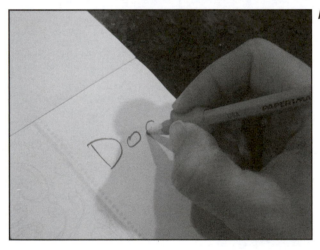

FIGURE 15-2

✦ Child picks up small, pellet-sized items (i.e., beads, small cubes, rice).
✦ Child uses tongs, chopsticks, or tweezers to pick up small objects. Suggested objects to pick up include marshmallows, Styrofoam, nuts, beads, and pom-poms. (Note that the closer to the tip the child holds the tong, the easier the activity becomes.)
✦ Child places toothpicks deep into resistive Theraputty to make a picture of a smiley face, a flower, a circle, etc. Child then removes each toothpick one at a time.

✦ Tissue paper projects: Child cuts up small strips of tissue paper. Child crumples each piece of tissue paper and then glues it to a paper to make a picture or create a letter of his/her name (Figure 15-3).

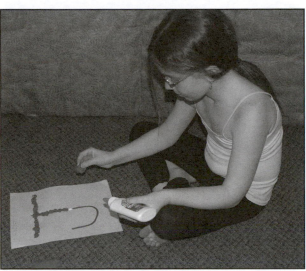

Figure 15-3

✦ Tissue paper butterfly: Child crumbles small pieces of cut-up tissue paper in each hand, holding hands in the air when crumbling and not against body. Child places pieces on a butterfly to decorate (Figure 15-4).

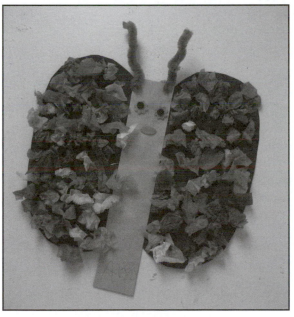

Figure 15-4

✦ String beads: Child laces beads to make a necklace. To downgrade this activity, the child can string beads onto a pipe cleaner instead of a string.

✦ Bead rolling: Therapist scatters beads on the table. Child picks up a bead one at a time and squeezes it between the index finger and thumb and holds for three seconds. Child then rolls bead back and forth, side to side, and then transfers it into a cup.

✦ Playdough rolling: child rolls pellet-size balls of playdough between the thumb and pointer finger, then squeezes them one by one using a pincer grasp.

◆ Small knobbed puzzles: Child holds the small knob on the puzzle piece to complete the puzzle (Figure 15-5).

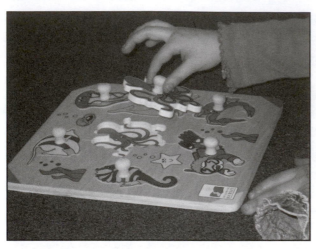

Figure 15-5

◆ Magna Doodle boards: Child holds the small tips of the Magna Doodle pieces to color a picture (Figures 15-6 and 15-7).

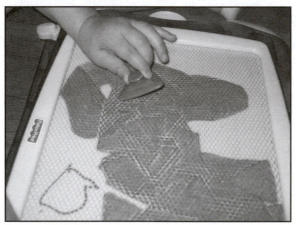

Figure 15-6

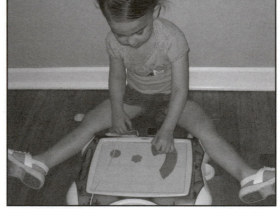

Figure 15-7

◆ Wind-up toys: Child winds up different wind-up toys and watches them go.

◆ Stamps: Child picks up different stamps with small handles and stamps a paper or own skin.

◆ Stickers: Therapist draws a picture of a smiley face or something else the child likes. Child puts very small stickers on the lines of the drawing and on the eyes, nose, mouth, etc.

Pincer Strengthening

✦ Child uses a reacher to pick up items off the floor and places them into a bucket (Figure 15-8).

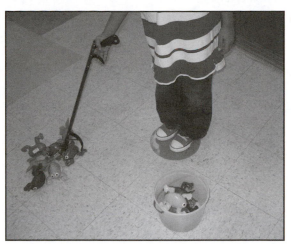

FIGURE 15-8

✦ Child completes clothespin activities, including:

⬦ Child places clothespins on string to make a necklace.

⬦ Therapist writes letters on clothespins and has child form words with clothespins (Figures 15-9 and 15-10).

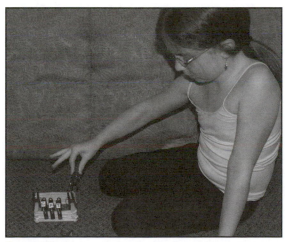

FIGURE 15-9

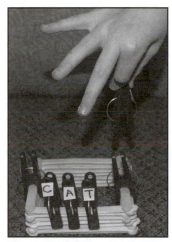

FIGURE 15-10

✦ Spray water bottles: Child helps water plants or washes off the chalkboard with a spray water bottle.

✦ Water guns: Therapist fills a water gun with water and creates a bull's-eye to be placed on the wall. Child stands a few feet away from the target and squirts the gun at the bull's-eye.

✦ Gluing activities: Child squeezes a glue bottle with the thumb and index fingers.

✦ Bubble wrap paper: Child pinches individual bubbles on bubble wrap paper between thumb and index finger.

✦ Sponge Activities:
   ✧ Child squeezes small sponges for sponge painting.
   ✧ Child wets small sponges and erases letters on a chalkboard (Figure 15-11).

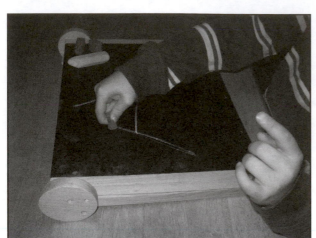

FIGURE 15-11

COMMERCIALLY AVAILABLE PRODUCTS

✦ "Operation" game
✦ "Squiggly Worms" game
✦ "Peg Domino"
✦ "Ants in the Pants" game
✦ "Design and Drill Activity Center"
✦ "Hungry Hippo"
✦ "Bed Bugs"
✦ "Plastic frog jumping toys"
✦ "Tiddlywinks"
✦ "Rock Em' Sock Em' Robots"

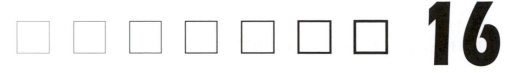

HAND STRENGTHENING

Proper hand positioning and acquired fine motor skills (as mentioned in previous chapters) are only part of what is needed for functional hand use. Hand strength is needed when lifting objects, grasping, and squeezing. Cutting, coloring, squeezing glue, and playing with playdough are different activities that require adequate hand strength.

Not only is hand strength important, but having endurance in the hand muscles is equally important. Children without proper endurance will struggle with writing a composition, coloring a worksheet, cutting out a picture, or any other prolonged fine motor activity. Many children with poor endurance are often aware of their limitations and commonly avoid fine motor activities, making it difficult to develop age-appropriate skills. This chapter will not only provide activities to increase hand strength, but also focus on endurance as an equally important principle.

Danto, A., & Pruzansky, M. *1001 Pediatric Treatment Activities:*
Creative Ideas for Therapy Sessions (pp. 125-130).
© 2011 SLACK Incorporated

Hand-Strengthening Activities

Push and Pull

+ Legos: Child pushes Lego pieces together tightly and then pulls them apart.
+ Pop beads:
  ◇ Therapist holds chain of pop beads and allows child to pull beads off the other end.
  ◇ Child pushes together pop beads and then pulls apart one bead at a time.
+ Rapper Snappers: Therapist crunches up a Rapper Snapper toy and holds one end while child grasps the other end. Therapist encourages the child to pull one way while the therapist pulls the other way. (The noise that this toy makes when being stretched is very reinforcing.)

Squeezing and Pinching

+ Tennis ball smiley face: To create this, the therapist or child draws a smiley face on a tennis ball and then an adult uses scissors or a knife to cut a 1-inch slit in the tennis ball over the mouth. Child then squeezes the sides of the tennis ball to place in small beads. After child completes placing the beads in ball, the child can make the tennis ball have a stomach ache and "throw up" all the beads (Figures 16-1 and 16-2). (The larger the slit on the tennis ball, the easier the activity.)

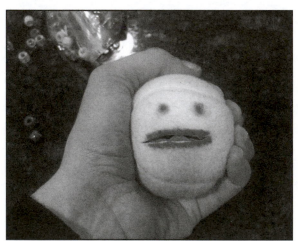

FIGURE 16-1   FIGURE 16-2

+ Theraputty exercises:
  ◇ Child pinches, pulls, and squeezes Theraputty.
  ◇ Child hides different objects in putty and then finds them as quickly as possible. (This activity can be made more exciting by using a timer to see how quickly child can work and then see if child can break his or her own record.)
+ Playdough:
  ◇ Child rolls and squeezes playdough.
  ◇ Child creates different objects with the playdough, including a ball, square, triangle, etc.
+ Knead dough: Child helps prepare dough for a baking activity and kneads dough until it is smooth.
+ Squeeze toys: Child squeezes a stress ball, Koosh ball, or another sensory ball.

✦ Using resistive grippers: Child performs hand-strengthening exercises on a hand gripper (Figures 16-3 and 16-4). Add rubberbands to increase resistance as needed.

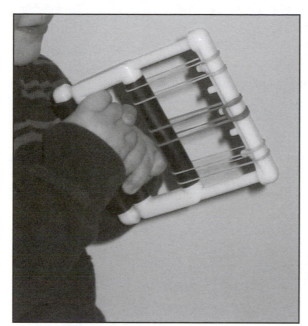

FIGURE 16-3

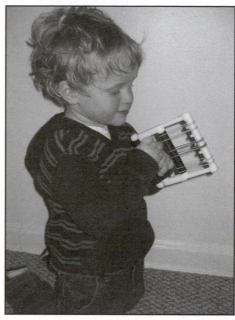

FIGURE 16-4

✦ Puff paint: Child squeezes puff paint onto a paper, a fabric, or another craft surface of choice to draw a picture or make a design.

✦ Squeezing glue: Child squeezes glue out of a container onto a line. (Be sure to use glue out of a container and not a glue stick.) This can be incorporated in to any gluing and pasting craft activity of choice.

✦ Child fills a squeeze toy with water and shoots it.

✦ Pustefix Bubble Bear: Child maintains a continuous squeeze on the bottle to keep the wand up out of the bottle and blows bubbles (Figure 16-5).

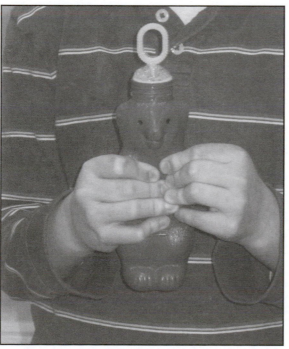

FIGURE 16-5

Increasing Endurance

+ Hand puppets: Child performs a play with different hand puppets.
+ Coloring: Child colors in large pictures in coloring books.
+ Snapping fingers: Therapist teaches child how to snap fingers together; they then snap along together to a song.
+ Hand exercises: Child opens and closes hand and fingers to the beat of a song.

Cutting Activities

+ Simple cutting: Therapist draws lines, shapes, or animals on a piece of paper. Child practices cutting along the lines in order to cut out the picture. (See Appendix pp. 217-222 for sample cutting handouts).
+ Snipping paper: Therapist holds a 1-inch strip of paper and allows the child to make snips in the paper (for lower level children).
+ Child performs resistive cutting activities:
    ◇ Child cuts strong Theraputty.
    ◇ Child cuts thick paper.
    ◇ Child cuts several papers at once.
+ Craft scissors: Child uses craft scissors to cut paper (craft scissors are more difficult to cut with than regular scissors.)

Pressing

+ Stapling: Child assists with stapling booklets of paper together.
+ Hole punching: Therapist draws a line or a shape onto a piece of paper. Child punches holes along the line so that the picture is "hole-punched" out of the paper (Figure 16-6).

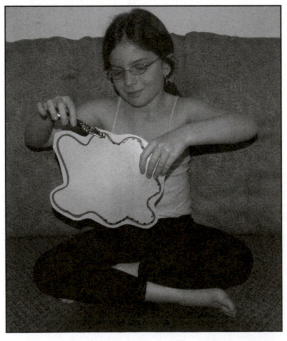

FIGURE 16-6

+ Child pops bubbles on bubble wrap paper, grabbing bubbles with whole fist.
+ Child presses down on pop-up toys (Figure 16-7).

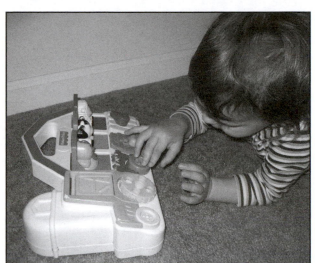

FIGURE 16-7

BODY STRENGTHENING AND STABILIZING

V

Having the skills and coordination needed to perform different activities throughout the day is only part of being successful with motor activities. It is critical that a child also has the necessary strength and stability. Strength and stability provide the foundation for movement and allow children to engage successfully and independently in daily living skills, sports activities, and academics.

This section will address different components of body strength and stability. The topics discussed include: core strengthening, balance activities, and activities to help improve shoulder and arm stability.

Core-Strengthening Activities

Core strengthening refers to strengthening the muscles in the trunk, stomach, and pelvic area. Decreased core strength will affect almost all fine- and gross-motor activities because the smaller muscles need to have a strong, stable core base from which to work. For example, when thinking about children with handwriting difficulties, many would assume there is some deficit or weakness in the hand. However, just as likely, there is decreased core strength and stability, thereby compromising the dexterity of the hand. While this is not always the case, weak core muscles are often the culprit for many fine-motor problems.

Core strength should be one of the first areas addressed when dealing with any fine-motor or gross-motor deficit. In this chapter, different core-strengthening exercises are provided that will help establish a strong foundation upon which to build further skills.

It is important that, when performing activities with infants, small children, and developmentally delayed children, the therapist be skilled in proper handling techniques, in order to safely and effectively implement the chosen activity. In order to become familiar with these handling techniques, the therapist should contact a trained pediatric occupational or physical therapist familiar with the specific population of interest.

Danto, A., & Pruzansky, M. *1001 Pediatric Treatment Activities:*
Creative Ideas for Therapy Sessions (pp. 133-146).
© 2011 SLACK Incorporated

Core-Strengthening Activities

Abdominal Exercises

✦ Modified sit-up: Place child on back on the floor or soft surface. Pull child's hands gently at the same time and let child use abdominal muscles to pull self to upright, seated position (Figure 17-1). (Developmental age 4 to 6 months.)

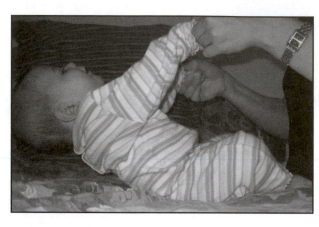

FIGURE 17-1

✦ "Row, Row, Row Your Boat" game: In this game, child sits on the floor, facing either therapist or another child, each holding onto one end of a jump rope (position I) or onto each other's wrists (position II). As both sing the song, one person leans back as the other leans forward and then the opposite.

 ◇ Position I (Figure 17-2).

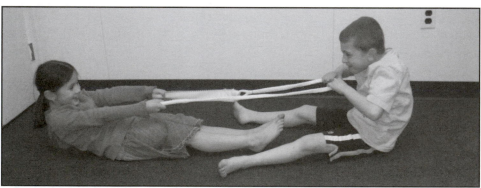

FIGURE 17-2

 ◇ Position II (Figure 17-3).

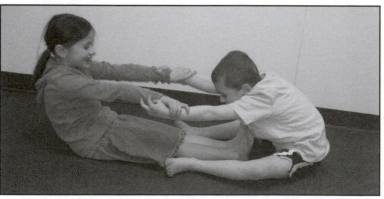

FIGURE 17-3

✦ Sit-ups and crunches: Child performs sit-ups and crunches on the floor. Therapist performs the same exercises with child in order to help continuously motivate child. (Developmental age 6 years and up.)

✦ Feet kick: Child lies supine (on back) on a mat with feet in the air. Therapist throws a large therapy ball towards child's feet. Child kicks ball upward and back toward therapist (Figure 17-4).

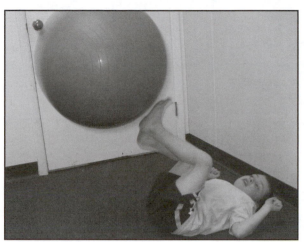

FIGURE 17-4

✦ Leg lifts: Child lies flat on floor and raises and lowers legs off the floor. (Developmental age 6 years and up.)

✦ Bicycle sit-ups: Child lies on back and brings the right elbow to the left knee, while extending the right leg. Then switches and repeats as tolerated (Figure 17-5). (Developmental age 6 years and up.)

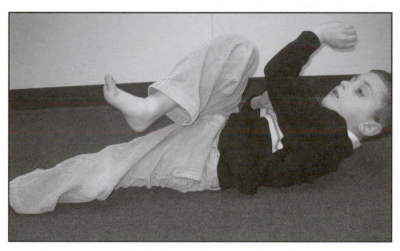

FIGURE 17-5

✦ Therapist lies on floor opposite child with therapist's feet touching child's feet. Therapist places a small ball between therapist's ankles and passes the ball to child. Child takes ball between child's ankles and passes ball back to the therapist in same way. This can also be played with two children (Figures 17-6 through 17-8).

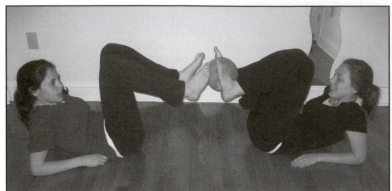

FIGURE 17-6

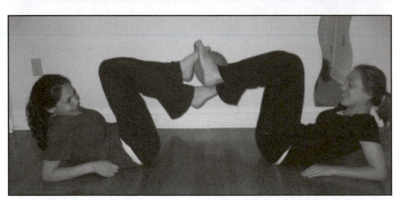

FIGURE 17-7

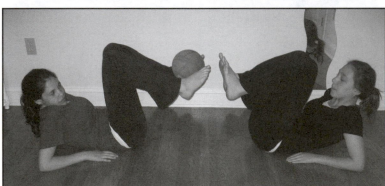

FIGURE 17-8

✦ Backward flip: Child lies on back on therapy ball. Child places arms on floor for support behind self. Child then flips body over (Figure 17-9).

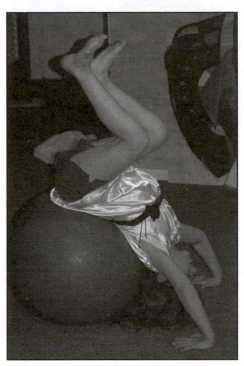

FIGURE 17-9

Whole Body Stabilization

✦ Sitting exercises (Developmental age 6 to 8 months.)

   ◇ The therapist places the child on the therapist's lap with the child facing the therapist. The therapist holds the child's hands and engages the child while the therapist lifts up one knee and then the other shifting the child's weight from side to side.

   ◇ Weight shifting: Therapist places child in sitting position on floor, providing minimal support. Therapist gently tilts child off balance to each side (one at a time) and then forward and backward. Therapist should try to only tilt the child slightly so that that child is able to regain balance and an upright, seated position independently when possible.

   ◇ Place child in sitting position for play and interaction with Boppy pillow around the child for support (Figure 17-10).

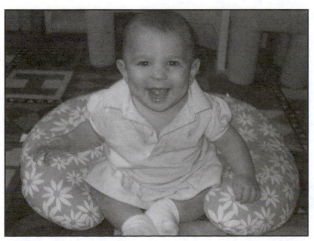

FIGURE 17-10

◇ Therapist places Hip Helpers on the child to give him extra support while sitting. Hip Helpers prevent the child from "w" sitting or sitting with legs spread wide apart, forming wide base of support, and "forces" the child to activate his/her trunk muscles while sitting (www.hiphelpers.com).

◇ Therapist places child in sitting position on the floor, providing minimal support as needed. Therapist has child stay in this position as tolerated while engaged in playful activities (Figure 17-11).

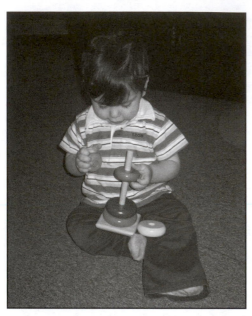

Figure 17-11

◇ While child is sitting, therapist holds a toy the child likes, such as a rattle, just above the child's head and encourages the child to reach for the toy. The therapist should have several different toys on hand so this can be repeated several times in a row.

◇ The therapist can place the toys on all different sides of the child so the child is required to reach in different directions to acquire the toys.

✦ Standing exercises: (Developmental age 3 to 4 months) (Cottrell, 2004, p. 20) Have child practice standing with limited support. Hold child under armpits (Figure 17-12) or by the hands (Figure 17-13), providing minimal support as needed. Place child's feet on a steady surface. Have child practice standing for several seconds at a time as tolerated.

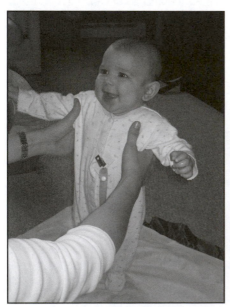

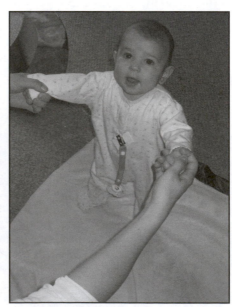

Figure 17-12   *Figure 17-13*

+ Kneeling activities: Child performs activities while kneeling on the floor (Figures 17-14 and 17-15). (While there are many games that can be played in this position, some ideas include: coloring activities, completing puzzles, playing catch, playing a card game on a low stool, and rolling a ring across the floor).

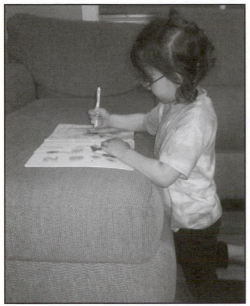

Figure 17-14

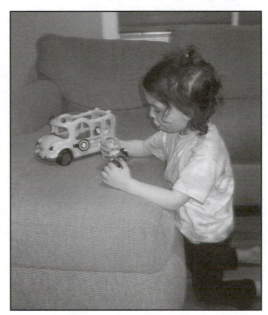

Figure 17-15

+ Child slowly walks up a ramp. Therapist makes sure child is standing upright and not using the hands or head to help climb.
+ Dizzy Disc: Child spins on the disc without falling off (Figure 17-16).

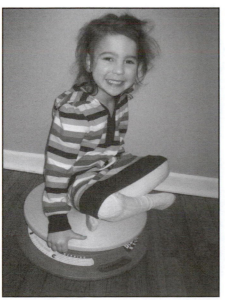

Figure 17-16

✦ Child sits on a bolster or peanut ball and reaches for far items placed on both sides. Child then throws the items into a basket (Figure 17-17).

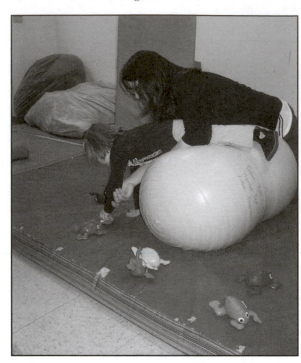

FIGURE 17-17

✦ Couch push-ups: Child lies prone (on the belly) on a couch, perpendicular to the length of the couch, with the upper body off the couch and hands on the floor and then performs push-ups (Figure 17-18). Child can also play a game or do a puzzle in this position.

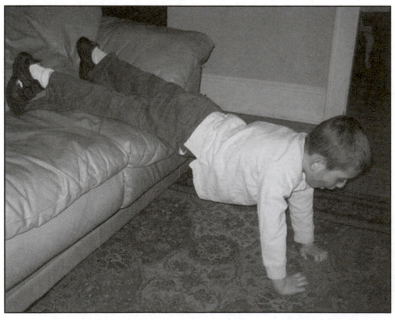

FIGURE 17-18

◆ Step-Ups: Child steps up and down from an object approximately 1 foot off of the floor. Therapist reminds child to place both arms out to the side when stepping onto and off of the surface in order to prevent the child from compensating by using arm muscles (Figure 17-19).

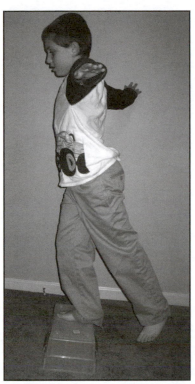

FIGURE 17-19

◆ Hippity Hop Toy: Child bounces across room on a Hippity Hop toy (Figure 17-20). (This toy can also be used as part of a relay race).

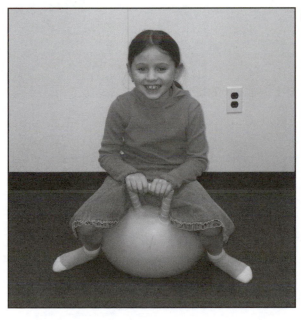

FIGURE 17-20

◆ Crab walking: Child crab walks across the room and picks up different objects along the way (Figure 17-21).

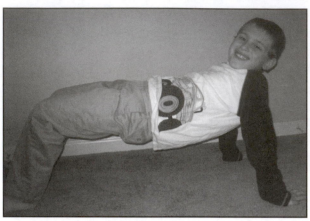

FIGURE 17-21

◆ Bridge making: Child lies on back on the floor. Therapist helps child make a bridge. Child then attempts to make a bridge independently (Figures 17-22 and 17-23). (Child can also make a bridge over a therapy ball.)

> *Increased caution should be taken with this activity, especially with children with lax ligaments or any medical conditions that may make them susceptible to dislocations.*

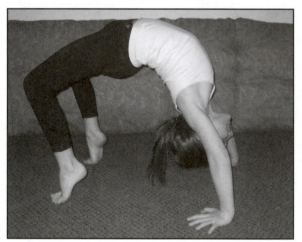

FIGURE 17-22

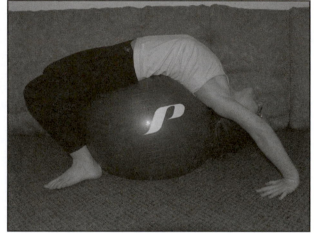

FIGURE 17-23

◆ Limbo: Child walks under a stick in the game of "Limbo." Therapist should ensure that child leans backward when walking under the stick and not forward (or else child will not be using abdominal muscles).

◆ Pogo Stick jumping: Child jumps across room on a pogo stick.

Suspended Equipment Activities

+ Therapist wraps child's legs around a T-swing. Child goes upside down and then tries to pull self up (Figure 17-24).

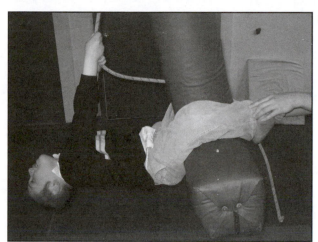

Figure 17-24

+ Log swing:
  ◇ Child straddles log swing and goes back and forth on moving swing without falling off.
  ◇ Child hangs upside-down on swing and holds on for a set count. Child then performs this activity several more times trying to beat own record for time held on (Figure 17-25). (This activity can be made more challenging by reaching for items on floor while hanging upside down.)

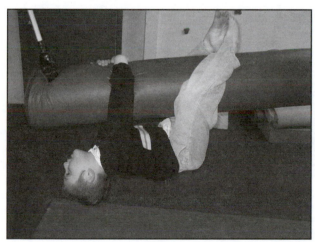

Figure 17-25

◆ Tire swing: Child straddles tire. Therapist makes sure child is not leaning forward or backwards, rather sitting upright so that the back and belly are not touching the tire. Therapist swings tire back and forth and side to side. Child holds on as long as possible (Figure 17-26).

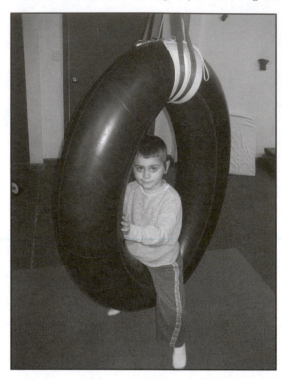

FIGURE 17-26

◆ Child hangs upside down on a trapeze bar and pulls self up (Figure 17-27).

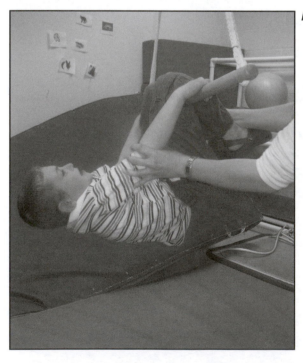

FIGURE 17-27

◆ Lycra swing: Child climbs up a long Lycra swing to the top and then slides down.

Therapy Ball Activities

♦ Child holds therapy ball against the wall only with the body (no hands). Child plants feet on floor and creates a bouncing momentum against the ball.

♦ Child holds a large therapy ball against the wall only with the body and then slightly moves the ball back and forth along the wall using his/her chest and stomach without using hands (Figure 17-28).

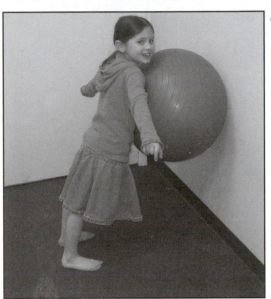

FIGURE 17-28

♦ Therapist places child in sitting position on therapy ball. While holding on to the child, the therapist rolls the ball forward and backward and side to side while engaging the child.

♦ Child lies on back on the floor and holds a therapy ball with both feet and hands. Therapist tries to gently pry ball away from child, while child tries to hold onto the ball (Figure 17-29).

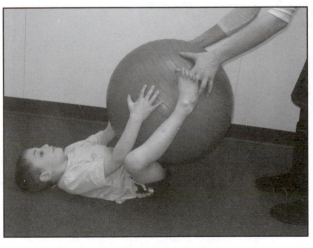

FIGURE 17-29

✦ Puzzle Ball sit-ups: Therapist scatters puzzle pieces around a therapy ball. Child sits on therapy ball and reaches for puzzle pieces placed behind or on the side of the ball. Child then performs a sit-up to put the piece into the puzzle frame (Figures 17-30 and 17-31).

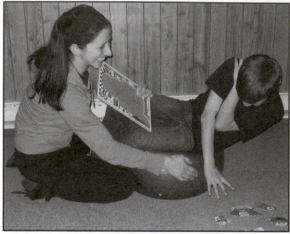

FIGURE 17-30

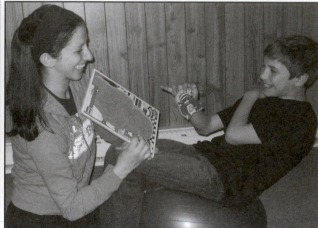

FIGURE 17-31

Climbing

✦ Climbing up furniture: Therapist brings child near a chair, couch, or small table. Therapist places a desired toy on the surface and encourages/assists the child, as minimally as possible, to transition from either sitting or quadruped to standing while holding on to the couch/chair, in order to reach for the toy (Figures 17-32 and 17-33).

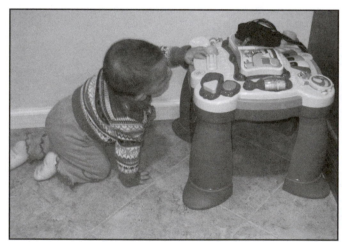

FIGURE 17-32

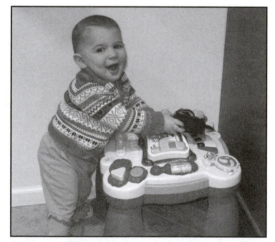

FIGURE 17-33

✦ Ladder climbing: Child climbs up a ladder or net in the therapy area or outside on the playground.
✦ Rock Wall games:
   ◇ Child climbs up the wall.
   ◇ Child climbs up rock wall, using only one specific color "rock."
   ◇ Therapist scatters rings on the top and along the rock wall. Child climbs across rock wall, picks up the rings, and throws them into a basket.

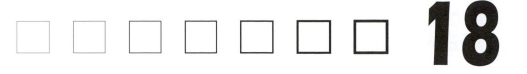

BALANCE ACTIVITIES

Balance is a necessary skill required for smooth and coordinated movement. Balance affects one's ability to walk, navigate through a messy room, climb steps, play, and perform other sorts of activities. In order to have adequate balance, one must first develop strong core muscles. In the previous chapter there are core-strengthening exercises. In this chapter, activities that work specifically on balance alone are provided.

While the act of balancing itself will help strengthen core muscles, this chapter was made independently of the previous chapter in order to highlight two main differences. The previous chapter has activities geared toward strengthening core muscles as a means for balance as well as other important skills for a child's development. Whereas in this chapter, improving balance is a goal in itself and additionally has an added benefit of strengthening core muscles in the process.

Specifically included in this chapter are balance activities that involve a child being on one foot or on unstable surfaces. The reason these activities are placed in this chapter is because a child exists in a dynamic environment. For example, a child will need to learn to walk on uneven sidewalks, up and down curbs, and over bumps on the grass. A child that is only able to maintain balance on stable and static surfaces would face serious difficulties in "real world" situations.

Additionally of significance in regard to balance are equilibrium reactions, body righting, and protective responses. In order to maintain balance, one has to be able to respond to external disturbances like being pushed or tripping over something. A normal response to these disturbances is with protective or equilibrium reactions. An equilibrium reaction is a reaction that occurs when one is tilted to one side and the body reacts by righting itself and tilting or leaning the body in the opposite direction. This reaction occurs in the frontward and backward, as well as in the lateral plane of movement. A protective reaction is used when one is falling and one "catches" oneself by stretching out one's arms in the direction of the fall. These reactions also occur in forward, backward, and lateral directions (Case-Smith, 2001). This chapter also provides activities that will help work on these reactions.

Danto, A., & Pruzansky, M. *1001 Pediatric Treatment Activities:*
Creative Ideas for Therapy Sessions (pp. 147-156).
© 2011 SLACK Incorporated

Balance Activities

One-Foot Activities

✦ Child maintains balance on one foot for X seconds and then alternates to other for X seconds.

✦ Child stands on one foot with other foot resting on a ball. Therapist stabilizes the ball if needed. To make activity more challenging, child performs an activity while on one foot, e.g., play catch, claps hands, etc. (Figure 18-1).

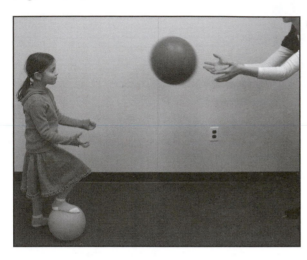

FIGURE 18-1

✦ Tapping cones with one foot: Child stands on one foot. Therapist places different numbered (or colored) cones on floor approximately one foot away from child. Therapist calls out a number (or color) and child taps the corresponding cone while maintaining balance (Figure 18-2).

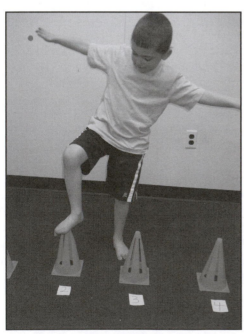

FIGURE 18-2

✦ Hopping activities:
   ✧ Child hops into rings placed on floor and freezes (Figure 18-3).

FIGURE 18-3

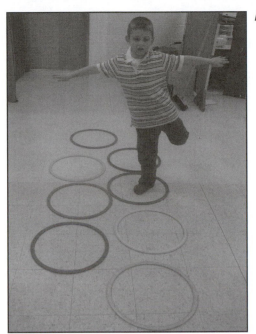

   ✧ Child hops over bumpy balance board sections (Figure 18-4).

FIGURE 18-4

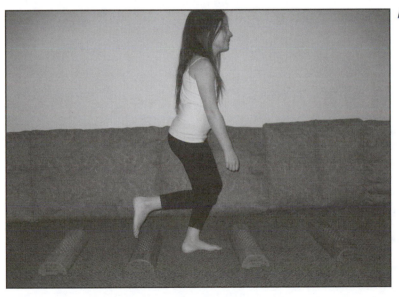

   ✧ Child hops in place.
   ✧ Therapist places laminated letters all around the floor. Child hops over the letters of child's name.

❖ Therapist places a rope on floor and tapes it down on both ends. Child hops over the rope and back (Figure 18-5).

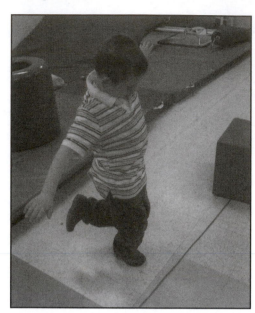

Figure 18-5

❖ Therapist places a rope on floor and tapes it down on both ends. Starting from one end of the rope, child hops over the rope, alternating landing on each side of the rope, making his way along the length of the rope as he is hopping, until he reaches the other end.

✦ "Balance on it": Therapist calls out a body part. Child balances on that body part. Some examples include right foot, left foot, both knees, one knee, both hands, etc.

Standing/Walking on Unstable Surfaces

✦ Balance board activities:
  ❖ Child steps on/off balance board.
  ❖ Child turns around in a 360 degree circle.
  ❖ Child plays catch with therapist.
  ❖ Child pops bubbles in air (Figure 18-6).

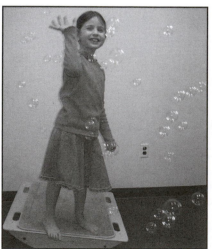

Figure 18-6

✧ Child reaches across midline for items in the air (Figure 18-7).

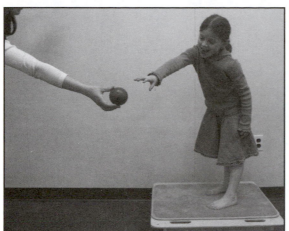

FIGURE 18-7

✧ Child plays basketball (Figure 18-8).

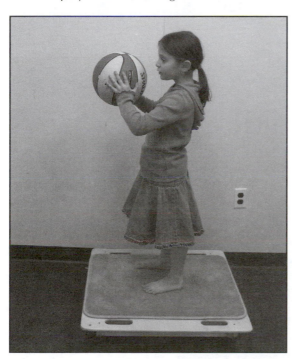

FIGURE 18-8

❖ Child throws a ball against a wall and catches it (Figure 18-9).

Figure 18-9

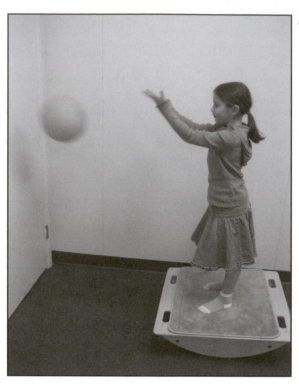

❖ Child places bean bag on head and balances it while on balance board.
✦ Balance beam activities:
  ❖ Child walks across balance beam.
  ❖ Child picks up items from the floor and throws them into target (Figure 18-10).

Figure 18-10

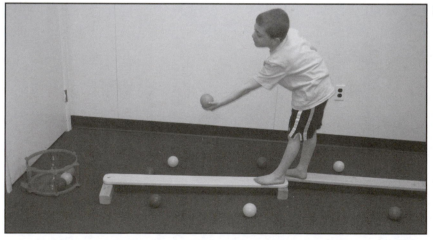

  ❖ Child walks across balance beam while holding an object in both hands.
  ❖ Child plays catch on balance beam.
  ❖ Child stands still, maintaining standing balance.
✦ Inflatable air disc: Child maintains balance with both feet placed on inflatable air disc.
  ❖ This activity can be downgraded by allowing child's toes to slightly slide forward and make contact with the floor (as opposed to being completely grounded on the air disc).

✦ Woggler: Child walks across the room on a Woggler (Figure 18-11).

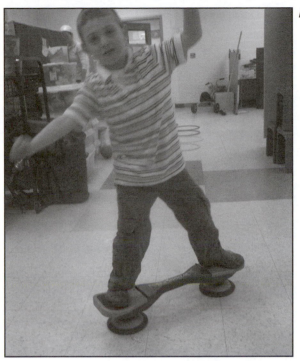

FIGURE 18-11

✦ Stepping stones: Child walks onto a specific colored or numbered stone (Figure 18-12).

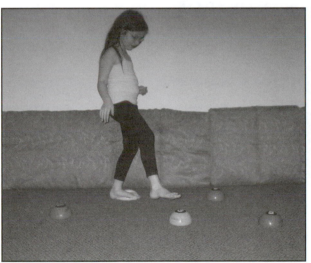

FIGURE 18-12

✦ Child walks on beanbags or other uneven surfaces (Figure 18-13).

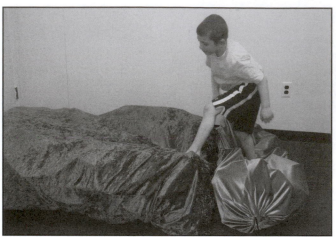

FIGURE 18-13

✦ Therapist places a therapy ball under a mat/ramp. Child walks up (Figure 18-14).

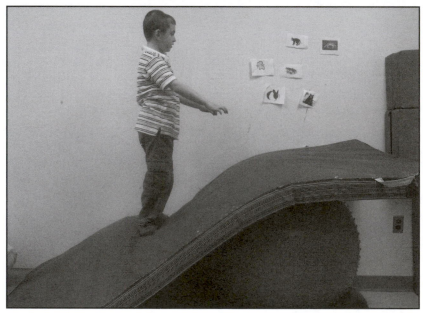

FIGURE 18-14

◆ Therapist places therapy ball under mat. Child "surfs" by balancing on moving mat and standing in one place (Figure 18-15).

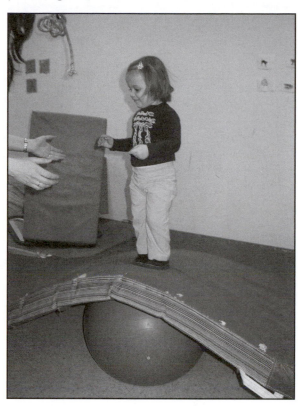

Figure 18-15

◆ Therapist places log swing on floor. Child walks across it without falling off. (Therapist may need to stabilize swing on the floor so it does not move around too much when the child is walking across it.)

◆ Curb walking: Child walks outside along the sidewalk curb.

◆ Walking on straight line: Child walks along a straight piece of long tape placed on the floor.

◆ Stair climbing:

   Must be done with close adult supervision

   ◇ Child walks up and down stairs without using railing.
   ◇ Child walks backwards up stairs and then down the stairs.

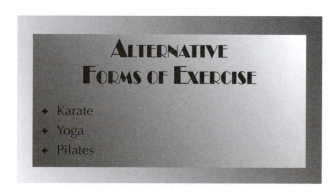

ALTERNATIVE FORMS OF EXERCISE

◆ Karate
◆ Yoga
◆ Pilates

Upper Arm Strengthening and Stabilization

Upper arm strength and stability are critical parts of functional hand use. As mentioned in the previous two chapters, core strength is a necessary prerequisite for fine and gross motor skills. Upper arm stability is the next required element in the hierarchy of hand function.

Children with poor upper arm strength and stability frequently have difficulty performing tasks with their hands. This is because they often exert excessive effort in order to fixate their arms and muscles during activities as a result of the decreased stability. When too much attention goes into trying to fixate and stabilize the arm, quality of work may suffer. The end result may be poor handwriting, inability to perform self-care activities, poor ball skills, and poor overall fine motor skills.

This chapter provides different activities to help strengthen and stabilize the arm and shoulder area. While the fun and engaging activities provided in this chapter can be performed in isolation, it would be most beneficial to follow up with a functional activity afterward.

Danto, A., & Pruzansky, M. *1001 Pediatric Treatment Activities:*
Creative Ideas for Therapy Sessions (pp. 157-172).
© 2011 SLACK Incorporated

Upper Arm Strengthening and Stabilization

Bearing Weight Through the Hands

✦ Place child in prone weightbearing position so that the child bears weight through forearms or hands. (Developmental age 4 to 6 months.)

✦ Lay on the floor next to the child, slightly higher than eye level. Alternatively, place child in prone position on a bed surface in order to make it easier for adult to be at child's eye level (Figure 19-1). (Developmental age 4 to 6 months.)

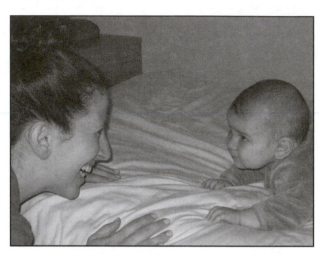

FIGURE 19-1

✦ Place child on "Boppy" or elevated surface in order to improve tolerance towards being in a prone position (Figure 19-2). (Developmental age 4 to 6 months.)

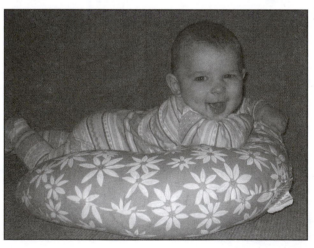

FIGURE 19-2

✦ Increase supervised "tummy time" activities for young children. (Developmental age 4 to 6 months.)

◇ Therapist lies at slight angle on floor, couch, or bed and places child on stomach/chest area in prone position (Figure 19-3).

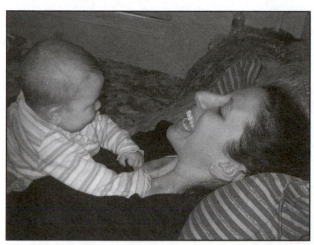

FIGURE 19-3

◇ Place a thin soft blanket on floor and place a toy in front of child on belly (Figure 19-4).

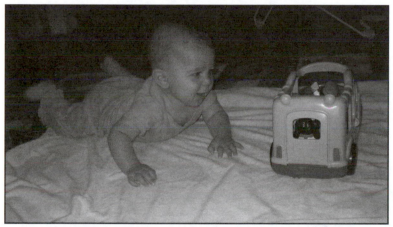

FIGURE 19-4

◇ Place child on stomach in front of a mirror.

◇ Place child on stomach over therapist's lap (Figure 19-5).

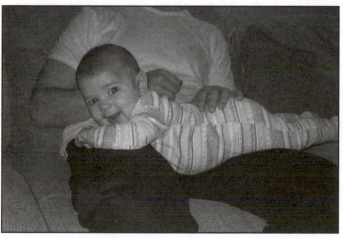

FIGURE 19-5

✧ Hold child horizontally in air, weight bearing on adult's forearm (Figure 19-6).

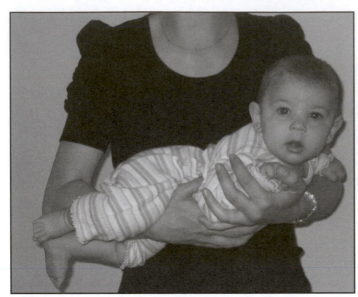

FIGURE 19-6

✦ Place child in quadruped position (Developmental age 7 to 10 months):

　✧ Have child maintain stationary position.

　✧ Have child reach for items from this position (Figure 19-7).

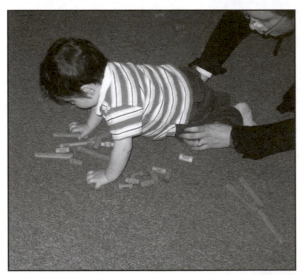

FIGURE 19-7

　✧ Have child go through crawling movements from this position with the therapist facilitating the movement.

♦ Child lies in prone position (on the belly) on a platform swing or a net swing a few inches off floor. Child leans over the edge so the chest is not on the swing, but rather off the edge. Therapist spreads out objects all around and under the swing. Child walks on hands to objects, picks them up, and throws them into a container, or performs another task with them (Figure 19-8).

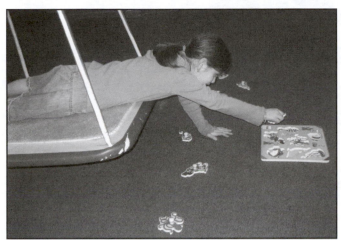

Figure 19-8

♦ Child lies prone (on belly) on a scooter board. Child holds onto a bungee cord or jump rope while being pulled by therapist.

♦ Child lies prone on a scooter board and propels self around the room in order to reach and pick up objects. For example, child picks up scattered bean bags or Koosh balls all over the floor and then places them into a bucket.

♦ Child walks feet up the wall while weight bearing through the hands on a mat (Figure 19-9).

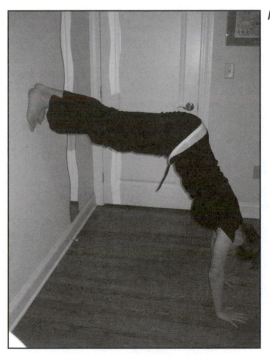

Figure 19-9

◆ Crab walking: Child walks in a supine (on back) position on hands and feet making sure that no other parts of the body are touching the floor (Figure 19-10).

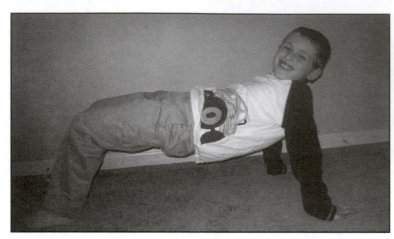

Figure 19-10

◆ Wheelbarrow walking:

   ◇ Child maintains a stationary wheelbarrow position.

   ◇ Child reaches for toys in this position.

   ◇ Child walks on hands with legs being held up in the air (Figure 19-11). (This activity can be graded by the distance walked and where the therapist places support when holding the child's legs. It is most physically challenging for the child when being held around the ankles. The closer to the hip the support is provided, the easier the activity for the child.)

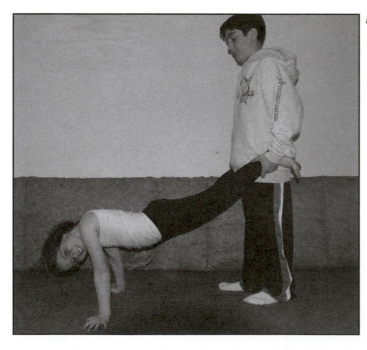

Figure 19-11

✦ Wheelbarrow walking races (Figure 19-12).

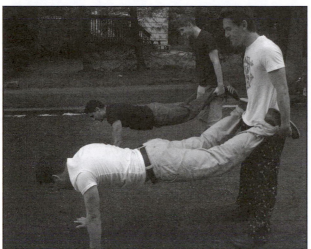

FIGURE 19-12

✦ Push-Ups: Child performs different push-ups including:
  ✧ Regular floor push-ups (Figure 19-13).

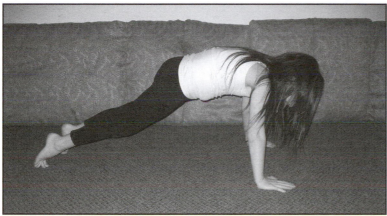

FIGURE 19-13

  ✧ Half push-ups with knees touching floor (Figure 19-14).

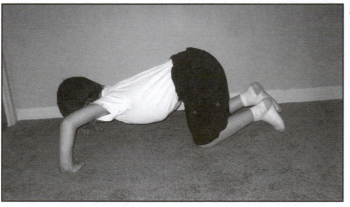

FIGURE 19-14

❖ Wall push-ups (Figure 19-15).

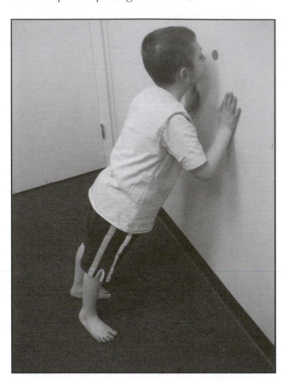

FIGURE 19-15

❖ Couch push-ups: Child lies on a couch on belly, hanging over the edge. Child places arms on the floor and pushes off the floor keeping lower body on the couch (Figure 19-16).

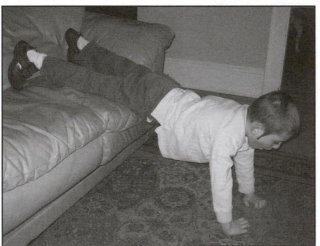

FIGURE 19-16

❖ Chair push-ups: Child sits on a chair, grabs each side of the chair with hands, locks elbows, pushes down, all while keeping bottom seated on chair (Figure 19-17).

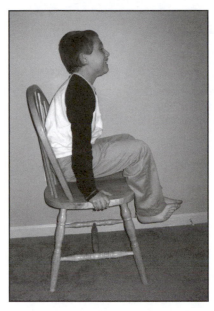

FIGURE 19-17

✦ Child leans over the edge of a solid stable surface, so that the chest is not supported by the surface. Therapist spreads puzzle pieces around the floor within arm's length. Child reaches for pieces and completes the puzzle (Figures 19-18 and 19-19).

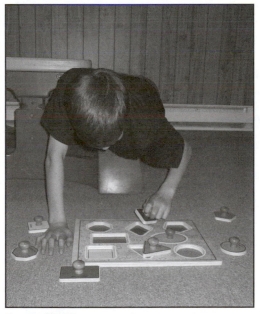

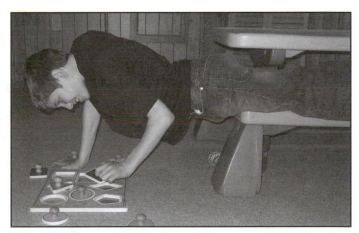

FIGURE 19-19

FIGURE 19-18

Using Vertical Surfaces

✦ Vertical surface writing:
   ❖ Child colors on an easel.
   ❖ Child writes on a chalk board.
   ❖ Child traces letters on a white board.

♦ Child completes writing sheets on a slant board.

♦ Child colors piece of paper taped onto the wall. (Child can color, paint, or write on this surface.)

✦ Child cleans off the chalkboard with an eraser or wet paper towel.

✦ Child pushes pegs into a peg board on vertical surface (Figure 19-20).

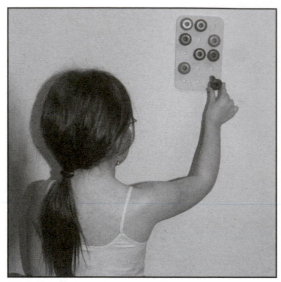

FIGURE 19-20

✦ Child places magnets on a vertical surface.

Stabilizing the Shoulder Against Gravity

✦ Child swings a jump rope.

✦ Child holds arms up in the air for X number of seconds.

✦ Child plays a game with magnetic fishing rods. Child uses the rod to lift up the fish when magnets connect (Figure 19-21).

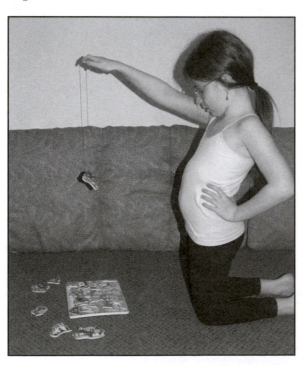

FIGURE 19-21

✦ Child builds a tower with blocks.

> *Note: This activity best works on shoulder stabilization when the height of the tower is above the child's shoulder level. This is so the child must reach up to place blocks on the tower.*

✦ Child lies prone on a platform swing. Child uses a reacher to pick up scattered beanbags/toys and places them into a bucket (Figure 19-22). (To upgrade or downgrade this activity, therapist can put the bucket at different heights and distances away from child.)

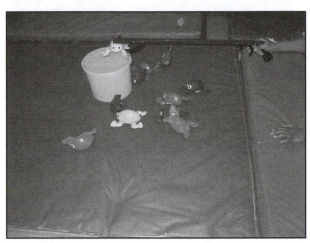

FIGURE *19-22*

Resistive Activities

✦ Child sits in a storage bin or barrel and pulls self out by climbing a rope that is being pulled tightly by therapist (Figure 19-23).

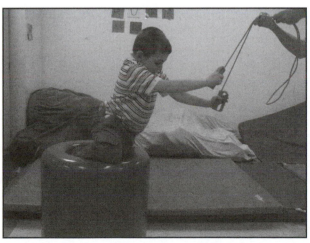

FIGURE *19-23*

✦ Child pulls apart Rapper Snappers or Therabands with arms straight out in front (Figures 19-24 and 19-25).

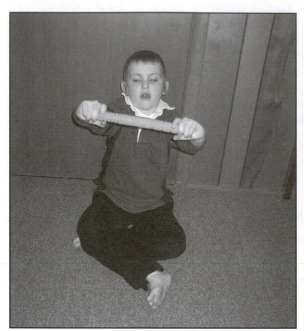

FIGURE 19-24   *FIGURE 19-25*

✦ Child places a mid-sized therapy ball between arms, not hands, and walks across the room holding the ball (Figure 19-26). (Use a smaller ball if this is too challenging.)

FIGURE 19-26

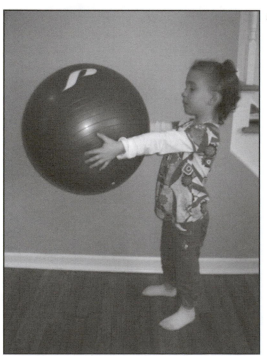

✦ Child climbs up a ladder.
✦ Child swings on a trapeze bar.

✦ Child swings across monkey bars in the playground (Figure 19-27).

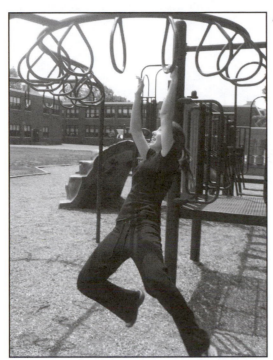

FIGURE 19-27

✦ Child hangs on monkey bar in place (Figure 19-28).

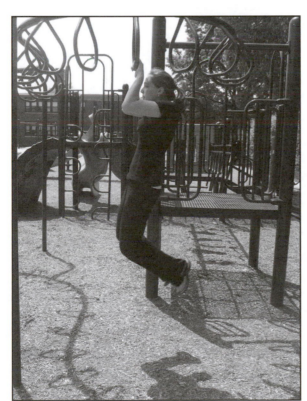

FIGURE 19-28

- Theraband exercises:
  - Child holds Theraband out in front of the body with both hands, pulls apart, holds, and repeats as tolerated (Figure 19-29).

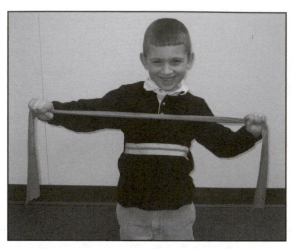

FIGURE 19-29

  - Child places Theraband behind the back with the Theraband wrapped around so child can grab it with each hand on both sides. Child straightens arms out to the side and holds. Repeat as tolerated (Figure 19-30).

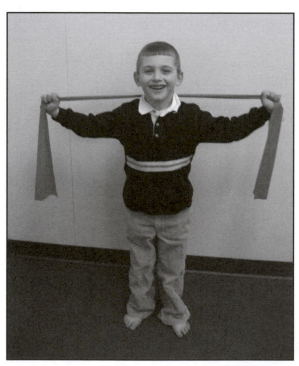

FIGURE 19-30

- Hula Hoop pulling: Therapist places child on a swing or a scooter while child holds onto a hula hoop. Therapist holds onto the other end of the hoop and pulls child around.

✦ Tug-of-war: This game can be played between child and therapist or between two children. This game should be closely supervised for safety concerns (Figure 19-31).

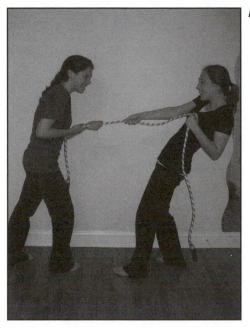

FIGURE 19-31

✦ Lifting weights: In a standing position, child holds weight in each hand at shoulder height with flexed elbows (Figure 19-32). Child fully extends arms and maintains shoulder flexion at 90 degrees. Repeat X number of times (Figure 19-33). (Repetitions should be determined by treating therapist.)

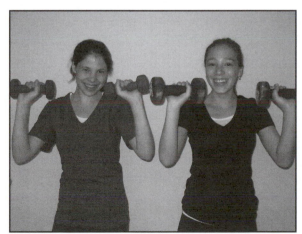

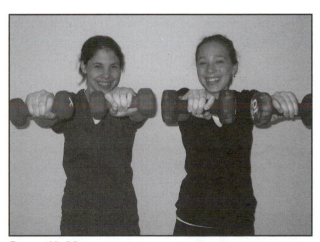

FIGURE 19-32   *FIGURE 19-33*

COMMERCIALLY AVAILABLE PRODUCTS

- ◆ "Lite Brite"
- ◆ "Fantacolor Jr."
- ◆ "Magnet Express"
- ◆ "Zoom Ball"
- ◆ "Jenga"
- ◆ "Melissa & Doug Magnetic Puzzles"
- ◆ "Don't Spill the Beans"

COGNITIVE AND HIGHER-LEVEL SKILL BUILDING

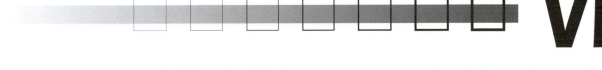

VI

Cognitive and higher-level skills are the skills that enable a child to perform executive functioning. Without these skills a child would not be able to answer a simple question, follow a multistep direction, or maintain focus during an activity. Children with poor higher-level skills and decreased cognition may appear disorganized and unfocused. A child with these difficulties may struggle to play a basic board game or engage in a simple ball game of toss and catch.

Included in this section are activities that will help improve overall organizational skills related to cognition and executive functioning. As described by Zeigler-Dendy (2002), components of executive functioning that impact school performance include the following:

✦ Working memory and recall (holding facts in mind while manipulating information; accessing facts stored in long-term memory).

✦ Activation, arousal, and effort (getting started; paying attention; finishing work).

✦ Controlling emotions (ability to tolerate frustration; thinking before acting or speaking).

✦ Internalizing language (using "self-talk" to control one's behavior and direct future actions).

✦ Taking an issue apart, analyzing the pieces, reconstituting and organizing it into new ideas (complex problem solving).

The specific areas of cognition and higher-level skill building that will be addressed in the upcoming chapters include increasing attention, increasing organizational skills, and improving social interaction and relatedness.

20

INCREASING ATTENTION

Being able to maintain attention is a prerequisite to engagement in any activity. There are two main types of attention that will be discussed in this chapter. The first form of attention is visual attention. This is the ability to visually attend to a task at hand. Many children do not look at what they are doing. When children do not look at what they are doing, they cannot be successful with almost any skills. For example, a child that does not look at his/her shoes cannot practice shoelace tying. A child that does not look at a piece of paper cannot improve handwriting skills.

The next level of attention that will be addressed in this chapter is the ability to maintain focus for more than a short period of time. This higher level of attention includes sustained attention and shifted/divided attention. Sustained attention refers to the ability to maintain attention on a specific point for an increased amount of time. Shifted/divided attention refers to the ability to move attention from one point to another.

The types of activities that will be suggested in this chapter are those that require continued engagement for a successful outcome. Most activities and games provided require both forms of attention. A therapist working with a child on these skills may downgrade the task by focusing on only one form of attention at a time. It is also up to the treating therapist to upgrade any activity provided as needed.

Other helpful strategies for increasing attention include the following:

+ A therapist should prepare the treatment area before treating a child in order to avoid having to stop an activity to obtain needed toys or materials.

+ Work and play in a tent/tunnel or cubicle in order to avoid outside distractions.

+ When working with a higher-level child, try working or playing with music on in background. This will help strengthen the child's ability to tune out extraneous background noise and focus on the demands at hand. This should only be done with a child who has already mastered the skill of being able to focus in a quiet and distraction-free environment.

+ Perform fast-paced activities in order to help the child stay focused.

Danto, A., & Pruzansky, M. *1001 Pediatric Treatment Activities: Creative Ideas for Therapy Sessions* (pp. 175-178).
© 2011 SLACK Incorporated

Activities To Increase Attention

Visual Attention

+ Therapist plays peek-a-boo with child.
+ Child bounces on a therapy ball or sits on an air disc while playing a game.
+ Child visually tracks an object in different planes. (Choose an object that is desirable to the child.)

Higher-Level Attention Building

+ Copy a pattern: Child laces beads in a pattern of colors or shapes.
+ Child colors lines on a paper in a specific pattern. Child repeats the pattern out loud in a sing-song way as a memory tool.
+ ABC wall game: Therapist places the letters A through E on the wall approximately half an inch apart in a random order. The letters should be large enough so a child can stand a few feet away from the wall and still see them. Child throws a ball at letter "A" and catches it. Child continues throwing it at the next letter and catches it. (Upgrade this activity by adding more letters or downgrade the activity by only placing two to three letters on the wall).
+ Child repeats a series of numbers, letters, or colors.
+ Board games: Therapist plays board game with child. Child attempts to remember when his/her turn is, without verbal prompting from therapist.
+ Child engages in different art and crafts projects.
+ Child sings parts of a song while performing an activity.
+ Child sings a complete song for therapist.
+ Freeze dancing: Child dances to music. When music stops, child freezes in place.
+ "Red light, green light, 1, 2, 3": Therapist stands next to the wall with back facing the child. Therapist says "red light, green light, 1, 2, 3" and then turns to face the child. Child runs to touch therapist, but stops once therapist turns around. If therapist catches child running, child must return to the wall and start again.
+ Child jumps into ball pit. Therapist instructs the child to throw balls into a basket in specific order, differentiating the balls by color. For example, therapist instructs child to throw "red, blue, red, yellow" in that specific order.
+ "Bingo": Child plays bingo in group or with therapist. (Can play this game with bingo cards with numbers, shapes, or pictures in order to upgrade or downgrade level of difficulty).
+ Card games: Therapist and child play card games together. Examples include gin, go fish, war, etc.
+ Memory/Concentration: Child and therapist play Memory and Concentration game together.
+ "I Spy": Therapist plays "I Spy" with child in a small room. (This will force the child to pay attention and look for details around the room in order to play successfully.)
+ "Arrow Game": Therapist hides something in the room or inside the building. Therapist tapes arrows (created out of masking tape) on the floor leading to the hidden toy. Child follows arrows and peels each arrow off of the floor as child passes each one.

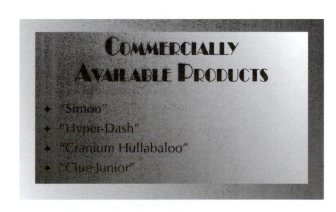

COMMERCIALLY AVAILABLE PRODUCTS

- "Simon"
- "Hyper-Dash"
- "Cranium Hullabaloo"
- "Clue Junior"

21

ORGANIZATIONAL SKILLS

Organizational skills are higher-level skills needed when organizing one's thoughts, following directions, problem solving, and strategizing. While the average person may take for granted organizational skills, these skills are not only needed during complex activities, but are also required for simple problem solving. Helping a child improve this set of skills will help open doors for a child. It will help increase the child's success and independence in numerous functional and academics areas.

This chapter provides different activities that must be upgraded or downgraded based on the child's functional level and abilities. If not properly graded, the child will either not be challenged enough or not be successful and only become frustrated. Demands placed on the child should be just slightly above the child's current ability, which research shows to be the optimal level for a child to learn. This level is called "the zone of proximal development," a concept developed by Russian psychologist Lev Vygotsky. This type of learning style enables a child to learn with assistance from someone more skilled than him or her and ultimately achieve independence in the skill (Vygotsky, 1986).

Danto, A., & Pruzansky, M. *1001 Pediatric Treatment Activities: Creative Ideas for Therapy Sessions* (pp. 179-182).
© 2011 SLACK Incorporated

Organizational Skills Activities

Following Set Directions

✦ Single step direction-following: Therapist creates a score sheet for child and gives him/her a sticker upon completing each direction correctly. (See Appendix p. 265 for sample sticker score card.) Single step directions can focus on commands with prepositional use. Examples include "Place the penny IN the box," "Stand ON TOP OF the paper," "Walk AROUND the chair," "Climb THROUGH the tunnel."

✦ Multiple step direction-following: Child follows a three-step direction. Example: "Run to the door, skip to the basketball hoop, and shoot three baskets." Therapist grades direction's level of difficulty based on child's ability.

✦ Child completes color by number/color by letter handouts. (See Appendix pp. 266-271 for sample handouts.)

✦ Child copies block or building designs.

✦ Child follows patterns with beads, pegs, or Froot Loops (Figures 21-1 and 21-2).

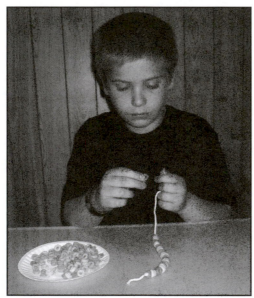
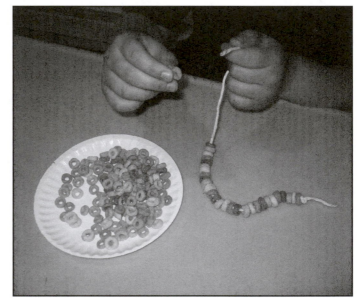

FIGURE 21-1   *FIGURE 21-2*

✦ Getting dressed: Therapist instructs the child to put on several articles of clothing in a specific order. For example, first socks, then shoes, then hat, then jacket, etc.

✦ Setting the table: Child follows either verbal or visual directions/instructions to set a table for meal time.

✦ Following a recipe:
   ◇ Child follows a simple cooking project from a ready-to-bake mix.
   ◇ Child follows a more difficult recipe from a cookbook, with assistance and supervision from the therapist as needed.

Strategizing

✦ Sudoku: This is a game that requires strategy and concentration. Visit www.websudoku.com to print out very simple forms of the Sudoku puzzles.

✦ Scavenger hunt: Therapist creates a list of items child must find in the room. Child checks off each item once it is found. (See Appendix p. 272 for sample scavenger hunt).

✦ Multi-step obstacle course: Child completes a series of tasks in an obstacle course. Some examples include climb through the tunnel, over the barrel, under the bean bag, jump into the hoop, walk around the cones, hop over the blocks, etc.

✦ Therapist tells child a letter. Child completes an obstacle course and at the end of the course finds the letter hidden among other letters hanging on the wall.

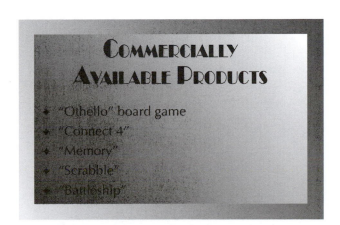

COMMERCIALLY AVAILABLE PRODUCTS

✦ "Othello" board game
✦ "Connect 4"
✦ "Memory"
✦ "Scrabble"
✦ "Battleship"

SOCIAL SKILLS

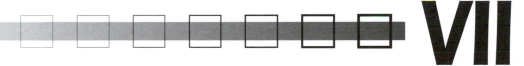

VII

Social skills refer to a set of skills that allow a child to act in a "socially acceptable" manner. While social skills come easy for some children, other children have difficulty in this area. Some children have difficulty playing cooperatively with other children, following rules when playing a game, conversing, answering questions, initiating appropriate conversation, regulating themselves in terms of body posture and physical proximity, and paying attention to their friends. They also often have difficulty reading facial expressions and picking up different nonverbal social cues. These difficulties may make it hard for a child to participate in classroom activities, play a game with peers, or maintain eye contact when speaking with a friend (Williamson & Dorman, 2002).

This section will help address social interactions and provide different games, group projects, group activities, and seasonal-based games and projects, all geared at improving social skills.

It is important to note that many of the activities provided work on multiple components of social competence and it is up to the therapist to choose which area to focus on and emphasize with a child.

INCREASING SOCIAL INTERACTION AND RELATEDNESS

Social interactions and social relatedness refer to a child's ability to interact and relate with other adults and children in the environment. Appropriate social interactions enable a child to make friends and create relationships with peers. Social interactions also help teach children how to behave in a socially appropriate manner.

There are different components that comprise appropriate social interactions and being related. Maintaining eye contact is one important part of being able to interact and relate with one's peers. Maintaining eye contact is often difficult, especially for children with an autistic spectrum disorder.

In addition to maintaining eye contact, there are also many other components of social competence that can be addressed while performing activities from this chapter. Some of these include reading facial expressions, understanding nonverbal social cues, maintaining appropriate personal space, modulating voice volume, having the ability to take turns, negotiating, and problem solving (Williamson & Dorman, 2002).

While there are an infinite number of games and activities that can be played to help work on increasing a child's social skills, this chapter will provide a sample of these sorts of activities. In this chapter are many games and activities that require pairing children into groups and require interdependence on the child's partner for success in an activity. The activities and games provided in this chapter should first be attempted with the child interacting with an adult. As the child comes closer to mastering an activity, he/she should then attempt the activity with another child.

Danto, A., & Pruzansky, M. *1001 Pediatric Treatment Activities: Creative Ideas for Therapy Sessions* (pp. 185-190).
© 2011 SLACK Incorporated

Increasing Social Interaction and Relatedness With Child and Peers

Back-and-Forth Games

✦ "Roly Poly": Therapist and child roll ball back and forth between them while sitting on floor with legs spread apart (Figure 22-1).

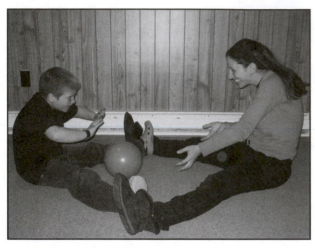

FIGURE 22-1

✦ "Wonder Ball"/pass the ball around game: Therapist and child pass ball back and forth between them while singing "Wonder Ball" song. When ball stops, child and therapist perform an action together (e.g., touch their heads, clap hands, etc.)

✦ Ball games: Child sits in a chair or stands in a barrel (in order to stay stationary) and plays toss/catch games with therapist (Figure 22-2).

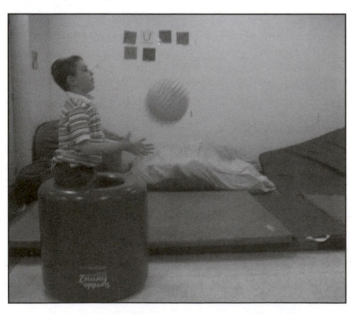

FIGURE 22-2

Interdependence Games

+ Peek-a-boo games: Child hides behind a pillow, under a small blanket, or in a tunnel and plays peek-a-boo with therapist.
+ Scooter-board games:
    ◇ Child sits on a scooter holding onto a rope. Therapist pulls child on scooter by pulling the rope.
    ◇ Two children sit on separate scooters. Therapist ties rope around the handle of two scooters. Two children hold hands while being pulled.
    ◇ Multiple children lie prone on scooter boards. Children make a train by holding onto the child's ankles in front of him/her. Therapist pulls rope tied onto the first scooter board.
+ Chasing games: Child and therapist play tag and other chasing games together.

Group Games

In the following games, it is important to determine the appropriate level of involvement of the therapist, whether it be directly playing, supervising, or facilitating.

+ Hide and Seek
+ Simon Says
+ Follow the Leader/Indian Chief
+ Hokey Pokey
+ Freeze dance
+ Musical chairs
+ "Red light green light 1, 2, 3"
+ Card games: Gin, War, Go Fish, etc.
+ Board games: Therapist chooses any board game that requires two or more players (Checkers, Candy Land, Guess Who? etc.).
+ Four corners: In this game one person is designated the counter. All four corners of the room are numbered corners one through four. The counter stands in the middle of the room and counts to ten, while covering his/her eyes. While the counter is counting, the other children can run around the room and pick one of the corners to be stand in. The counter then calls out a number between one and four, referring to one of the corners with his/her eyes still closed and then opens his/her eyes. All of the children who are standing in the corner called out are out. Counter repeats counting until only one child is left. The last child left wins and gets to be the counter in the next round.

Sensory Activities With Movement, Touch, and Song

+ "Ring Around the Rosie."
+ "This Little Piggy…" (Figure 22-3).

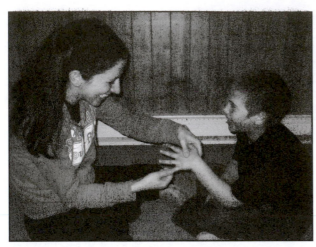

FIGURE 22-3

+ "Patty Cake," "Miss Mary Mack" (Figure 22-4).

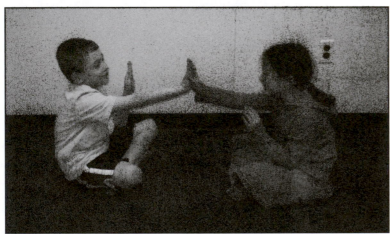

FIGURE 22-4

+ Hot potato (Figures 22-5 and 22-6).

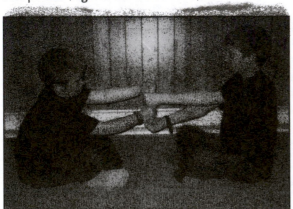

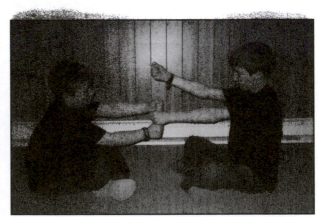

FIGURE 22-5

FIGURE 22-6

◆ "Itsy Bitsy Spider": Therapist sings song with child while trying to make eye contact.

◆ "If You're Happy and You Know It": Therapist sings this song with child. Child finishes each phrase and acts it out with therapist. For example, "If you're happy and you know it… touch your nose."

◆ Therapist places child on swing and says "go" and "stop" when starting and stopping movement. Therapist attempts to have child say these words in order to direct therapist to move swing. Therapist can also try to have the child count "1, 2, 3" in order to direct therapist to swing the swing.

◆ Therapist places child on a therapy ball. Therapist bounces child on the ball while focusing on eye contact and increasing vocalizations and other sounds.

◆ Therapist provides linear vestibular movement on a platform swing while maintaining eye contact with child.

Making Eye Contact

◆ Therapist plays games with child in front of a mirror and makes eye contact through the mirror. For example, therapist and child sing "Head, shoulders, knees and toes."

◆ Copy games: Child watches therapist and:
  ⋄ Imitates different facial expressions.
  ⋄ Imitates a beating pattern on a drum.
  ⋄ Imitates different funny body postures.

◆ Facial cues: Therapist makes different faces at child. Child tells therapist what emotion is being displayed (anger, sadness, happiness, surprise, etc.). Child then tries to imitate a specific emotion.

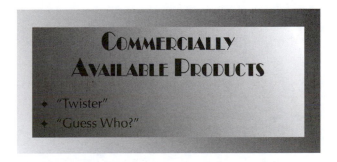

COMMERCIALLY AVAILABLE PRODUCTS

◆ "Twister"
◆ "Guess Who?"

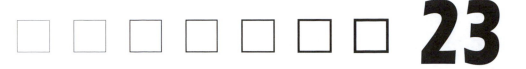

GROUP ACTIVITIES

Group activities are a great way to help build social skills and friendship among children of all ages. Fun and exciting games and projects that can be played with two or more children are provided in this chapter. The treating therapist can choose to have the listed activities played between multiple children or between therapist and child. Some children with more severe social deficits will often require an adult to heavily prompt and guide them during many of the social activities provided.

When planning a group, it is important to understand the population one is working with and to know any specific child's needs in advance. This is to ensure there will be adequate adult supervision and assistance. A group's success is often dependent on adult supervision and assistance.

Danto, A., & Pruzansky, M. *1001 Pediatric Treatment Activities:*
Creative Ideas for Therapy Sessions (pp. 191-202).
© 2011 SLACK Incorporated

Group Activity Themes

Funny Ball Games

✦ Over/under game: Children line up and pass a small ball between them. The first child passes it backwards over his/her head and the next one passes it backwards between the legs. Once the last child gets the ball, all the children turn and face the opposite direction and play again (Figures 23-1 and 23-2).

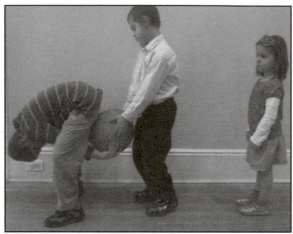

FIGURE 23-1

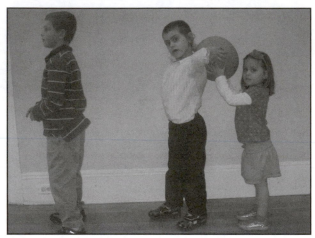

FIGURE 23-2

✦ Funny passing game: Children sit in a circle and try to pass a small ball without using their hands. They can pass it by grabbing it with their elbows, feet, knocking it with their heads, or any other safe and creative way.

✦ Neck ball: Children pass a small ball from one child to the next without using hands and passing it only with their necks (Figure 23-3).

FIGURE 23-3

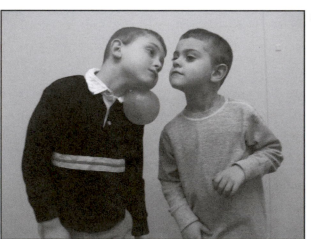

Color-Themed Groups

+ "Color Hokey Pokey": Therapist cuts out strips of tissue paper and gives children different colored strips. Children then sing the "Hokey Pokey" song: "Put your red hand in, etc." After this is done with tissue paper, it can also be done with small balls or different colored bean bags.

+ Therapist covers a flash light with different pieces of colored cellophane wrap. Therapist shuts the lights and shines each color on the ceiling and then has each child find one item in the given color. Children bring item into the middle of the circle.

+ Color hunt: Children close their eyes and pick a small piece of colored construction paper out of a bag filled with pieces of construction paper in various colors. Children each try to find something of that color in the room.

+ "If You're Wearing….": Play a "Simon Says" style game. For example, "If you're wearing red, stand up. If you're wearing blue, clap your hands. etc."

+ Color association game: Therapist places index cards with different colored fruit, animals, clothing, etc., on a board in front of the children. Children take turns sorting objects into the correct color category.

+ "I Spy": Children play the "I Spy" game using colors as clues. For example, therapist says, "I spy something red that is on the top shelf of the bookcase." Children then try to guess the chosen object.

+ Building a colored tower: Children pick a color out of a hat and then add the corresponding colored block to a tower. Children see how tall they can make the tower before it falls.

+ Child picks a color out of a hat and then hops/jumps/wheelbarrow-walks to something matching the corresponding color across room.

Letter-Themed Groups

+ Therapist places several index cards with letters on a wall, orienting the cards in different directions (some cards will be upright, upside-down, sideways, diagonal, etc.). Therapist chooses a random word. Child throws a ball against the wall onto the first letter of the word and then catches it as it bounces back. Child continues to throw the ball against the wall onto the second and then remaining letters of the word and then catches it.

+ Letter-themed obstacle course: Child picks a letter out of a hat and looks at it, but therapist holds onto it. Child then completes the obstacle course. At the end of the obstacle course several letters should be hanging on a wall either in the same case or in a different case (upper or lower). Child identifies the chosen letter on the wall and then tapes it on top of the matching letter on the wall (Figure 23-4).

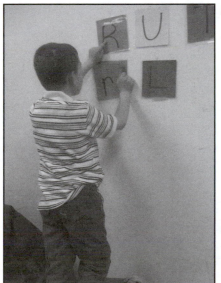

FIGURE 23-4

◆ Each child builds the letters of his/her name out of pegs. Therapist mixes all the assembled letters together and spreads them out on the floor. Each child individually walks to find the letters of his/her name and then spells it out on a table (Figures 23-5 and 23-6).

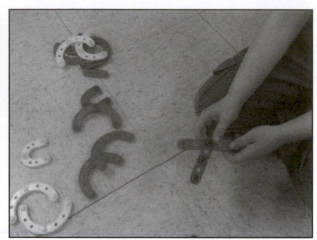

FIGURE 23-6

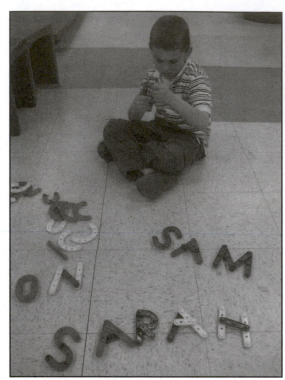

FIGURE 23-5

Number-Themed Groups

◆ Children go outside and collect small leaves or flowers on the ground. Children are given a picture of an empty tree or flower. Children then glue the leaves or flower petals onto the page. Children count up the number of leaves/petals on the tree or flower and write that number on the tree trunk/flower stem (Figures 23-7 and 23-8).

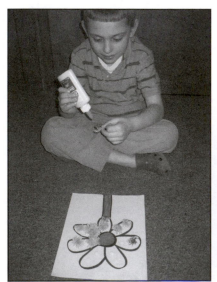

FIGURE 23-7

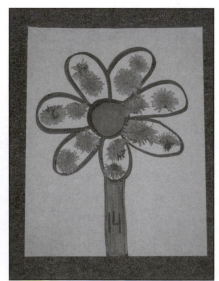

FIGURE 23-8

✦ Number chart: Children are given the number chart (see Appendix p. 273) and then asked to glue the corresponding number of sequins or foam pieces onto the row (Figures 23-9 and 23-10).

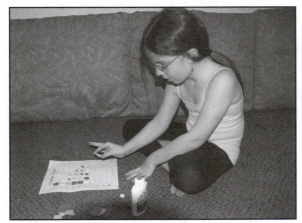

FIGURE 23-9

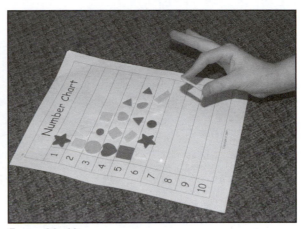

FIGURE 23-10

Shapes Groups

✦ Therapist places different shapes all over the floor around the room. Therapist gives the children gross motor instructions regarding the shapes. For example, say, "Jump over the squares, hop over the triangles, march around the rectangles, etc."

✦ Therapist sticks different shaped items in a bag (square book, triangle puzzle piece, ball, etc.). Children stick their hands into the bag and use stereognosis (the ability to identify objects based on touch without the assistance of vision) in order to determine what shape they are touching.

✦ Children make shapes out of a jump rope (Figure 23-11).

FIGURE 23-11

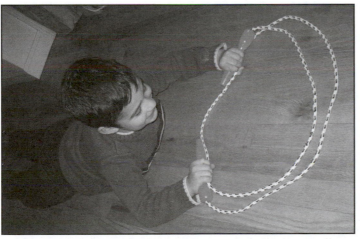

✦ Children try to make shapes with their fingers. Children then lie on the floor and position their bodies to make specific shapes. Therapist takes a picture with a Polaroid or digital camera of the children once they are in the correct position.

✦ Shape instructions: Therapist provides each child with shape handout (see shape instruction handout in Appendix p. 274). Children follow the key at the bottom of the page. Instructions include make dots in the circles, make vertical lines in the triangles, and make horizontal lines in the squares.

✦ Shape collage: Therapist takes a piece of paper and makes large circles, squares, rectangles, and any other shape all over the paper. Therapist gives out craft foam pieces. Children glue the corresponding shapes into the large shapes on the paper (Figure 23-12). An alternative activity would be to have the children just draw smaller shapes into the large ones (Figure 23-13).

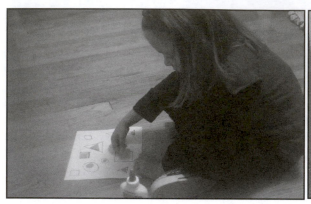

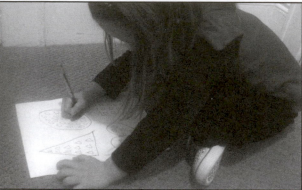

FIGURE 23-12   *FIGURE 23-13*

✦ Children create pictures solely out of cut out shapes (e.g., of a person, house, ice cream cone, etc.; Figure 23-14).

FIGURE 23-14

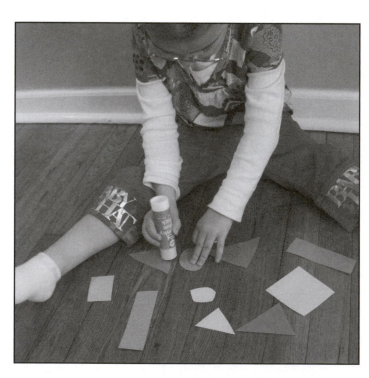

Teamwork Games

✦ Relay races: Examples include three-legged race, potato sack race, place a spoon in mouth with an egg or ping pong ball on the spoon, transfer water from one bucket to another, frog jump, backward walking, twirling, etc.

✦ Clothing race: Therapist places different articles of oversized clothing on one side of the room. Children must race to the other side of the room and get dressed in the large T-shirt, shorts, and socks as quickly as possible (Figures 23-15 and 23-16).

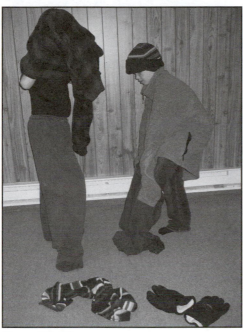
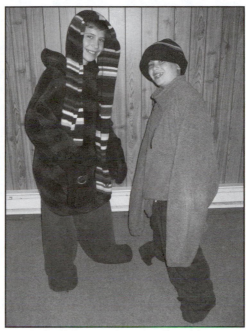

FIGURE 23-15   FIGURE 23-16

✦ Scavenger hunt: Children play the game together as a group in a circle. Child gets a turn to find one item on the list and bring it back into the circle. Alternately, small groups can be made and the children can play in teams against one another. (See Appendix p. 272 for a sample scavenger hunt.)

Social Skill Building

✦ "Get to know you game": Children are given the empty sticker chart. (See Appendix p. 265 for the sticker chart). Each child picks a random category out of a bag with a question on it. Child then asks one friend in the circle the answer to this question. For example, if the category picked is favorite colors, child must ask someone in the circle, "What is your favorite color?" and then be able to tell the group the answer. For each correct question and answer, both children are given a small sticker to place on the sticker chart.

✦ Mummy wrap: Children pair up in teams of two or more people. One child is designated to be the "mummy." The mummy must stand still while other children in group wrap toilet paper around him/her.

✦ Human puppet game: Therapist pairs up children. Therapist places large pieces of paper on floor. One child from each pair lies on paper. Other child traces out the body outline. Children then switch. After completed, children cut out their puppets (with therapist assistance, if needed), draw or glue on body parts, and decorate them (Figures 23-17 and 23-18).

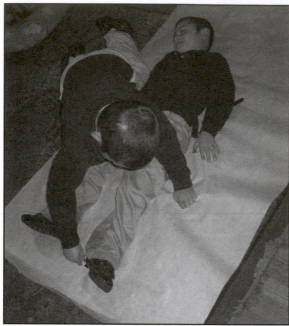

FIGURE 23-17

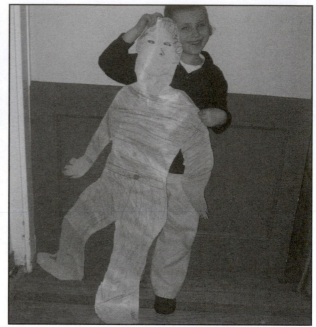

FIGURE 23-18

✦ Children make hand puppets out of brown paper bags. Children glue on googly eyes, color in mouth, put on feathers for hair. Children sing songs and talk to each other using their puppets (Figure 23-19).

FIGURE 23-19

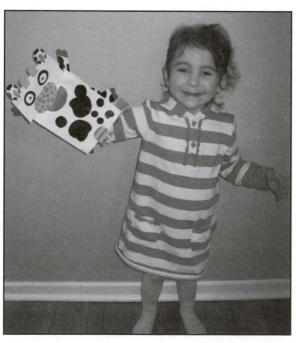

◆ "Bridge-Body-Connect"

    ◇ Several children perform a bridge with their backs (therapist assistance may be required). Remaining children crawl under all of the other children's bridges (Figure 23-20).

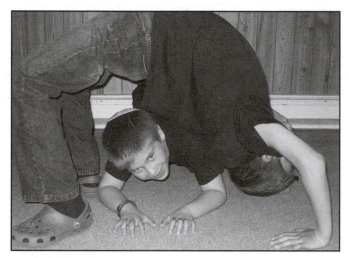

FIGURE 23-20

    ◇ Therapist then pairs up the children in groups of two. Children lie on their backs on the floor with their feet touching their partner's feet. Both children raise their legs off of the floor and press their feet against their partner's feet (Figure 23-21). Remaining children crawl under the bridge.

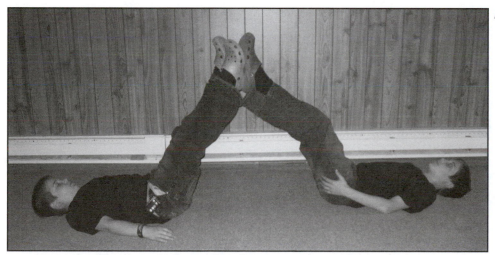

FIGURE 23-21

    ◇ Children then face each other and hold hands. Children raise their hands so other children can climb under. (Think of other fun and creative ways to connect the children's bodies and make more bridges.)

◆ Telephone: Children sit in a circle. One child or therapist whispers a word or sentence into the next child's ear. That child whispers what he/she heard to the next child. Finally, the last child says what he/she heard out loud and the original person says whether or not that was correct.

◆ Cookie making: Therapist takes cookies and has children spread icing on them with their fingers. Children then decorate with sprinkles, small pretzel pieces, raisins, etc. Each child makes two cookies, one for themselves and one for a friend.

◆ "Ring Around the Rosie"

◆ Rolling game: Children all lay on a mat on their backs next to each other. Sing the song, "There were (insert number) children in a bed and the little one said roll over." Children continuously roll without touching the child next to them while singing the song and freeze once they reach the edge of the mat. Children then continue rolling the other way on the mat.

Groups to Work on Attention and Organization

✦ Random association groups: Children match pictures or words to something associated with it (e.g., summer/hot, dog/bone, bed/pillow, raindrop/umbrella, etc.).

✦ Association groups based on seasons and holidays. Therapist creates cards with association pictures/words. Children play matching and sorting games with cards.

✦ Memory/Concentration: Children play memory/concentration games in a group.

✦ Bingo: Children play bingo together. Children can use numbers, shapes, or pictures in bingo. Therapist can create bingo sheets with a few items on the page, or many, in order to upgrade or downgrade the level of difficulty.

Sensory Groups

✦ Sensory baseball: Child comes up to bat either on a tee or be thrown a slow pitch. Child hits the ball and runs around the bases. Each base should be a sensory activity. For example, first base could be a trampoline that you have to jump on ten times. Second base could be a large bean bag that the child crashes into. Third base could be a wedge that child must crawl up and jump off, etc.

✦ Oral motor group

  ◇ Therapist places a pom-pom on the table. Children blow the pom-pom back and forth between them without letting the pom-pom fall off the table (Figure 23-22).

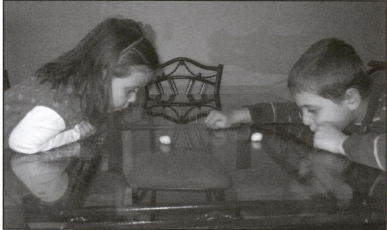

FIGURE 23-22

  ◇ Children can also each be given whistles and take turns blowing them. After this, the therapist can hold an empty paper towel roll and sing a song through it (using it as a microphone). Therapist should only start the song and the children should pass around the "microphone" and take turns saying the specific verse in the song.

✦ Pin the Tail on the Donkey: Children can play this game with eyes open, closed, spinning, and no spinning.

✦ Parachute games: Children walk holding onto parachute handles, run underneath parachute when it is raised, sit on the middle of parachute, and be pulled by therapists (Figure 23-23).

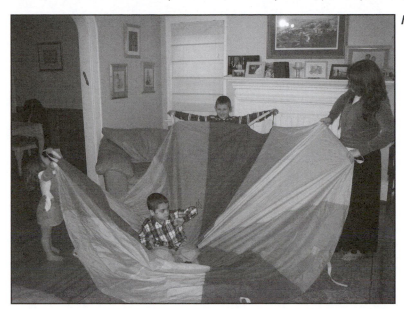

FIGURE 23-23

✦ Parachute popcorn game: Children crumple large strips of tissue paper and throw them into the middle of the parachute. Once all the colors are in the middle, children swing the parachute up and down and watch the "popcorn." Try to keep the popcorn from falling off the sides as long as possible (Figure 23-24).

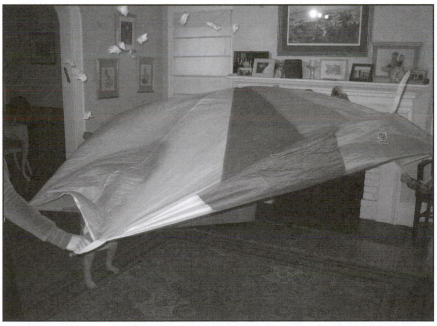

FIGURE 23-24

SEASONAL-THEMED PROJECTS AND ACTIVITIES

The different seasons are a time for learning and fun. Children are often highly motivated to engage in seasonal-themed projects and activities. In this chapter are different activities and projects that can be completed during the different seasons. When selecting a project or activity, it is important to keep in mind the child's abilities and the specific skills that need to be strengthened before selecting an activity.

Because many teachers and therapists work with a variety of children from different backgrounds, it is important to keep in mind cultural and religious sensitivities before selecting a project or activity.

Danto, A., & Pruzansky, M. *1001 Pediatric Treatment Activities: Creative Ideas for Therapy Sessions* (pp. 203-208).
© 2011 SLACK Incorporated

Seasonal-Themed Projects and Activities

Fall Activities

✦ Games:

  ❖ Pin the stem on the pumpkin: Draw a very large pumpkin without a stem on a piece of oak tag or large paper. Cut a stem out of green construction paper. Place adhesive on the back of the stem. Blindfold the children and have them take turns trying to place the stem on the correct spot on the pumpkin. (Same rules as "pin the tail on the donkey.")

  Therapist must use sound judgment when selecting blindfold activity with a specific child and must carefully supervise any activity involving blindfolding.

  ❖ Apple bowling: Place a picture of apples on bowling pins. Have the children roll a ball and try to knock over the pins. (If bowling pins are not available, small cones can be used.)

  ❖ Fall bingo: Create a fall bingo sheet. Sample categories can include apples, pumpkins, acorns, leaves, pinecones, and trees with fall-colored leaves. Have children play bingo in a group together.

  ❖ Fall memory: Create small cards with fall-themed pictures. Make two of each. Mix the cards together and place them faced down on the table. Then have the children play fall memory. (Sample categories are included in fall bingo activity).

  ❖ Turkey hunt: Make photocopies of a picture of a turkey. Hide the turkeys around the room and have the children find the hidden turkeys. After one round, have the children split into two groups. Have one group of children hide the turkeys and then allow the other group to search for the hidden turkeys (then switch hiders and finders groups.)

  ❖ Fall gross motor activity: Create two sets of matching fall cards (sample categories provided above in fall bingo). Spread the two piles on opposite sides of the room. Instruct the child to pick a specific card from the first pile and then have the child go the other pile while performing a gross motor instruction (e.g., hop, jump, skip, gallop, wheelbarrow walk, crab walk, scooter, backward walk, frog jump, etc.).

  ❖ Leaves hunt: Go outside and search for different types of leaves.

  ❖ Visit the Web site http://www.dltk-holidays.com/. You can automatically create bingo sheets, memory cards, and other holiday-themed games.

✦ Projects:

  ❖ Cut out and color pumpkin shapes. Then hide the pumpkins around the room and have a pumpkin hunt where the children must find their friends' hidden pumpkins.

  ❖ Tissue paper corn project: Create a corn template and have children cut it out. Have long pieces of green tissue paper and small pieces of yellow tissue paper. Have children glue on the long green pieces for the husk. Then have children take one yellow piece of tissue paper in each hand and crumple them up. Glue the yellow tissue paper pieces in the middle for the kernels. Continue crumpling and gluing until the entire template is covered with tissue paper.

  ❖ Scarecrow project: Give each child five different pieces of a scarecrow that have to be put together in the correct order. Each child should be given a cut-out pumpkin head, straw body, pants, shoes, and straw hat. (The body parts can also be photocopied and then the children can cut the parts out by themselves.)

  ❖ Acorn maracas: Have children collect acorns from outside. Color and decorate two paper plates. Staple the plates together with the tops of the plates facing each other. Do not staple all the way around so there is some space left with a hole to put in the acorns. Give each child acorns and have them put the acorns inside the hole. Then staple the plates all the way so there is no space for the acorns to fall out. The children can play with and shake their maracas to the beat of a tune.

  ❖ Pumpkin decorating: Provide small pumpkins to the different children and allow the children to decorate the pumpkins with markers, paint, sequins, feathers, and other crafts.

❖ Hand turkeys: Trace each child's hand on brown construction paper to make a turkey. Glue feathers onto the finger tips and a googly eye onto the thumb.

❖ Fruit turkeys: Place an orange or an apple sideways on the table. Place four toothpicks on the top of the fruit and one toothpick into the side of the fruit. (The toothpicks will serve as feathers and the head.) Stick four raisins into each toothpick on the turkey's back and one grape on the turkey's head. Then place one mini-marshmallow on the top of each of the four toothpicks on the turkey's back.

❖ Thankful turkey project: Have the children glue colorful tissue paper onto the back of a paper plate, which will serve as the turkey's back. Give each child four pieces of construction paper that have been cut into the shapes of turkey feathers. Have the children write one thing on each feather that they are thankful for. Then glue the feathers onto the plate. Place googly eyes for the eyes, and draw on a nose.

❖ Book of thanks: Have the children create a "book of thanks" by writing a different word or sentence on each page about something they are thankful for. Then have the children illustrate their "book of thanks." In order to bind the pages of the book together, punch holes on the edge of the paper and then tie string or yarn through it. (The books can also be stapled together.)

❖ Hand trees: Therapist paints child's arm and hand with brown and green paint respectively. Child presses down on paper to form the trunk and leaves of the tree. Child dips fingertips into paint of the different fall colors. Child then makes dots on paper to finger-paint leaves all over the tree.

❖ Leaf shading: Collect leaves from the ground. Place the leaves under a piece of white paper. With a crayon, color lightly on the paper over where the leaf was placed. The shape of a leaf will appear on the paper.

Winter Activities

◆ Games:

❖ Visit the Web site http://www.dltk-holidays.com/. You can automatically create bingo sheets, memory cards, and other holiday-themed games.

❖ Bundle up the bear: To work on dressing skills, have a child dress a stuffed animal with winter clothes, using infant's clothing. It can be made into a game of "we pass the bear around" and each time the bear stops, another article of clothing is added.

❖ Indoor sledding: Have child sit on a scooter-board while holding onto a jump rope with two hands, an adult or another child can pull the rope to propel the child around the room.

❖ Winter bingo: Create a winter bingo sheet. Sample categories can include snowman, sled, jacket, ice-skating, skiing etc. Then have children play bingo in a group.

❖ Winter memory: Create small cards with winter-themed pictures. Make two of each. Mix the cards together and place them faced down on the table. Then have the children play winter memory. (Sample categories are included in winter bingo activity.)

◆ Projects:

❖ Snowman: Make a snowman using three small-sized, white paper plates. Cut out an orange triangle for the mouth, glue on buttons for the eyes, and use crumpled tissue paper balls to form the mouth. Staple on brown pipe cleaners for the arms.

❖ Snowflake projects: Fold a white paper in half several times, then snip different shapes with a scissor. Unfold the paper to see the snowflake. It can be decorated with glitter for a sparkle effect.

❖ Handprint evergreen tree with snow: Therapist paints green finger paint on child's hands. Child makes multiple upside-down handprints on a large paper in the shape of an evergreen tree (triangle). A triangle border can be drawn on the paper prior to the painting if necessary for the child. Therapist then makes a mixture of half glue/half shaving cream. Child paints mixture on tree to get a puffy "snow" effect when dry.

❖ Create calendars: Have children draw a picture associated with each month of the year. Print out the 12 months of the year. Place picture above each month and staple calendar together.

Spring Activities

- ✦ Games:
  - ❖ Children each go into potato sacks and pop up and down out of the potato sack pretending to be flowers blooming. Children then have a potato sack race.
  - ❖ Flowers memory game: Create flower memory cards by coloring matches of different sorts of flowers on the cards. Then have the children play a game of memory.
  - ❖ Visit the Web site http://www.dltk-holidays.com/. You can automatically create bingo sheets, memory cards, and other holiday-themed games.
- ✦ Projects:
  - ❖ Pop up ground hog on a popsicle stick: Print out picture of groundhogs. Have child color them and glue them to a popsicle stick to make a puppet. Cut out two squares of brown paper and staple them together on two opposite sides (leaving the top and bottom open). Put the puppet into the "pocket-under ground" and then make it pop up.
  - ❖ Make bunnies: Create a blank template of a rabbit on a piece of construction paper. Have the children place small pieces of Styrofoam or crumpled white and pink tissue paper on the bunny. Then make the mouth and whiskers with black pipe cleaners (Figure 24-1).

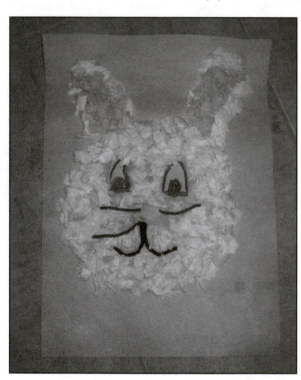

FIGURE 24-1

  - ❖ Bunny hats: Cut out hats with bunny ears and place on the children's heads. Then have the children hop around the room like bunnies.
  - ❖ Tissue paper flowers: Cut four to six pieces of tissue paper into 8 x 10-inch pieces. Place the pieces on top of each other and fold the pieces like an accordion. Tie the center of the folded tissue paper with a green pipe cleaner. Then slowly unravel each layer, one at a time creating the flower's petals.
  - ❖ Flower vases: Children paint and decorate empty water bottles or seltzer bottles with sequins. Children can also wrap different yarn or string around bottles.

❖ Paper plate picture frames: Have children bring in a picture with his/her mother. Have the children cut a hole in the center of the plate slightly smaller than the picture. It may be helpful to trace a line for the children and start the first cut so the child does not rip the paper. Have the children decorate the plates with glitter, stickers, sequins or other craft materials. Last, have an adult staple the picture onto the plate from behind (Figure 24-2).

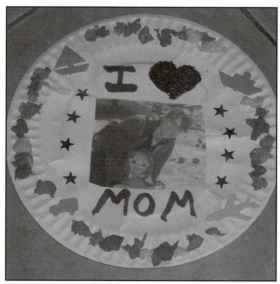

FIGURE 24-2

Summer Activities

✦ Games:

❖ Summer bingo: Create a summer bingo sheet. Sample categories can include American flags, barbecues, hot dogs, hamburgers, ketchup, grills, fireworks, beach, sun, swimming, suntan lotion, ice cream, etc. Then have children play bingo in a group.

❖ Summer memory: Create small cards with summer-themed pictures. Make two of each. Mix the cards together and place them face down on the table. Then have the children play summer memory. (Sample categories are included in summer bingo activity.)

◆ Projects:

   ◇ American flags: On a white paper draw an American flag template. Cut out red strips and glue them to every other stripe. Cut out a blue square for the corner and use either small star stickers or silver glitter for the stars (Figure 24-3).

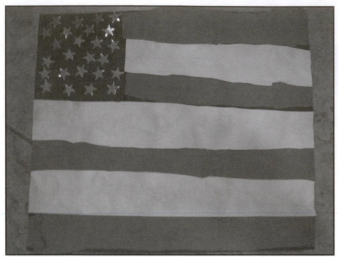

Figure 24-3

   ◇ Water-colored fireworks: Provide each child with different colored paint in cups. Have the children squeeze the paint from the cup into a medicine dispenser and then create droplets on a white piece of paper. Then have the children blow through a straw onto the paint droplets to create fireworks.

   ◇ Glitter fireworks: Have children glue shooting lines onto a black piece of construction paper and then sprinkle glitter onto the lines (Figure 24-4).

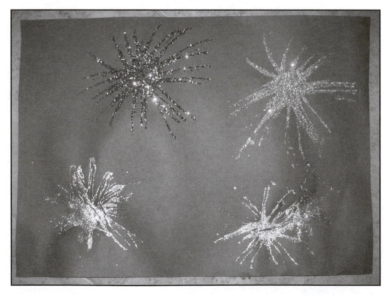

Figure 24-4

   ◇ American flag safety pin: Place small red, white, and blue beads onto the safety pin in the pattern of the American flag.

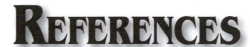

REFERENCES

Ayres, A.J. (1965). Patterns of perceptual-motor dysfunction in children: A factor analytic study. *Perceptual and Motor Skills, 20,* 355-368.

Ayres, A.J. (2005). *Sensory integration and the child. Understanding hidden sensory challenges.* Los Angeles, CA: Western Psychological Service.

Beery, K.E., Buktenica, N.A., & Beery, N.A. (2010). *The Beery-Buktenica developmental test of visual-motor integration* (6th ed.). San Antonio, TX: Pearson.

Case-Smith, J. (2001). *Occupational therapy for children.* St. Louis, M.O.: Mosby, Inc.

Cottrell, R.P.F. (2004). *National occupational therapy certification exam review & study guide.* Evanston, IL: International Education Resources.

Giroux Bruce, M.A., & Borg, B. (2002). *Psychosocial frames of reference.* Thorofare, NJ: SLACK Incorporated.

Hammill, D., Pearson, N., & Voress, J. (1993). *Developmental test of visual perception* (2nd ed., DTVP-2). Austin, TX: Pro-Ed Inc.

Martin, N.A. (2006). *Test of visual perceptual skills-non motor* (3rd ed.). Novato, CA: Academic Therapy Publications.

Parham, D.L., & Fazio, L.S. (1997). *Play in occupational therapy for children.* St. Louis, MO: Mosby Inc.

Raghavan, P., Krakauer, J., Santello, M., & Gordon, A. (2007). Relationship between finger individuation and shaping the fingers to object contours. *American Journal of Physical Medicine & Rehabilitation, 86,* No.4, 327.

Reichow, B., Barton, E., Neely Sewell, J., Good, L., & Wolery, M. (2010). Effects of weighted vests on the engagement of children with developmental delays and autism. *Focus on Autism and Other Developmental Disabilities, 25,* 3-11.

Danto, A., & Pruzansky, M. *1001 Pediatric Treatment Activities:*
Creative Ideas for Therapy Sessions (pp. 209-210).
© 2011 SLACK Incorporated

Rosenfeld-Johnson, S. (2001). *Oral-motor exercises for speech clarity.* Tuscon, AZ: Innovative Therapists International.

Takata, N. (1974). Play as a prescription. In M. Reilly (Ed.), *Play as exploratory learning* (pp. 209-246). Beverly Hills, CA: Sage Publications.

Tecklin, J.S. (2008). *Pediatric physical therapy (*4th ed.). Baltimore, MD: Lippincott, Williams, and Wilkins.

VandenBerg, N.L. (2001). The use of a weighted vest to increase on-task behavior in children with attention difficulties. *American Journal of Occupational Therapy, 55,* 621-628.

Van Hof, P., Van der Kamp, J., Savelsbergh, G.J.P. (2002). The relation of unimanual and bimanual reaching to crossing the midline. *Child Development, 73,* 1353-1362.

Vygotsky, L. (1986). *Thought and Language.* (Rev. ed.). Cambridge, MA: The Massachusetts Institute of Technology.

Wilbarger, P., & Wilbarger, J. (1991). *Sensory defensiveness in children aged 2-12: An intervention guide for parents and other caretakers.* Santa Barbara, CA: Avanti Educational Programs.

Williamson, G.G., & Dorman, W.J. (2002). *Promoting social competence.* Austin, TX: Hammill Institute on Disabilities.

Zeigler-Dendy, C. A. (2002, February). 5 components of executive function and a bird's-eye view of life with ADD and ADHD: Advice from young survivors. *CHADD ATTENTION Magazine.*

APPENDIX

Danto A., & Pruzansky M. *1001 Pediatric Treatment Activities: Creative Ideas for Therapy Sessions* (pp. 211-274).
© 2011 SLACK Incorporated

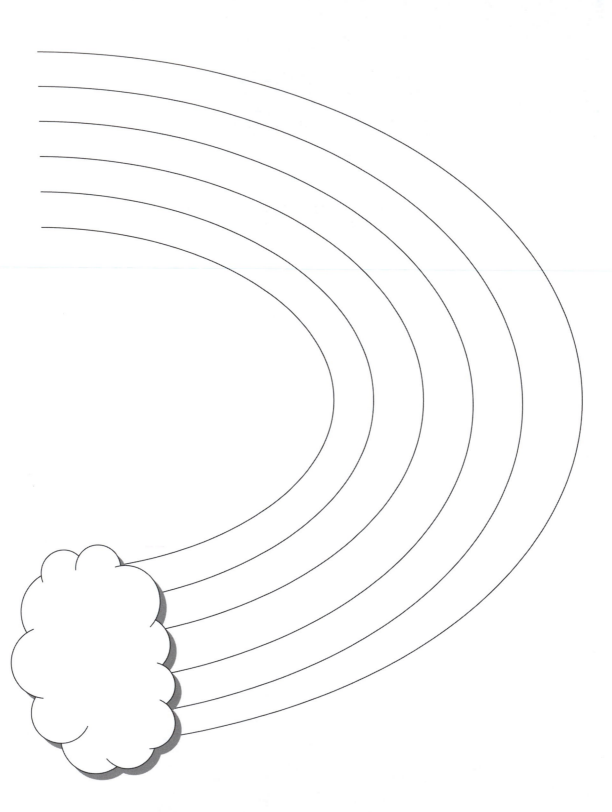

From Danto A., & Pruzansky M. *1001 Pediatric Treatment Activities: Creative Ideas for Therapy Sessions*. Thorofare, NJ: SLACK Incorporated; 2011.

Cut out the boxes and then sort the following shapes from biggest to smallest.

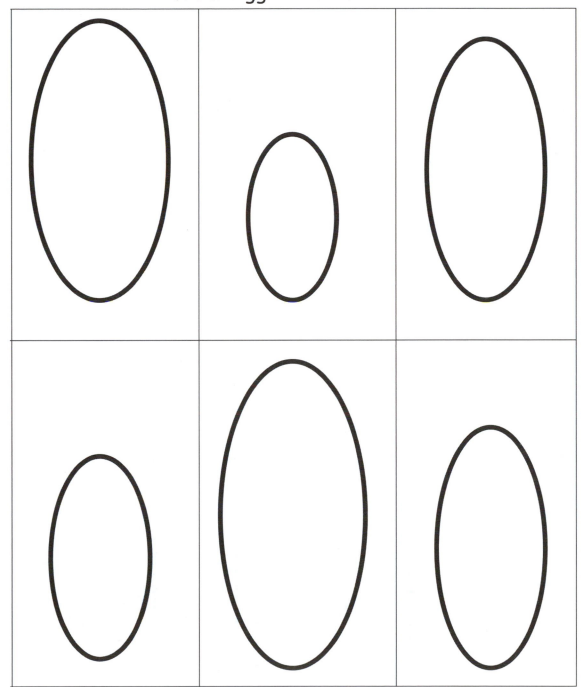

Cut out the boxes and then sort the following shapes from biggest to smallest.

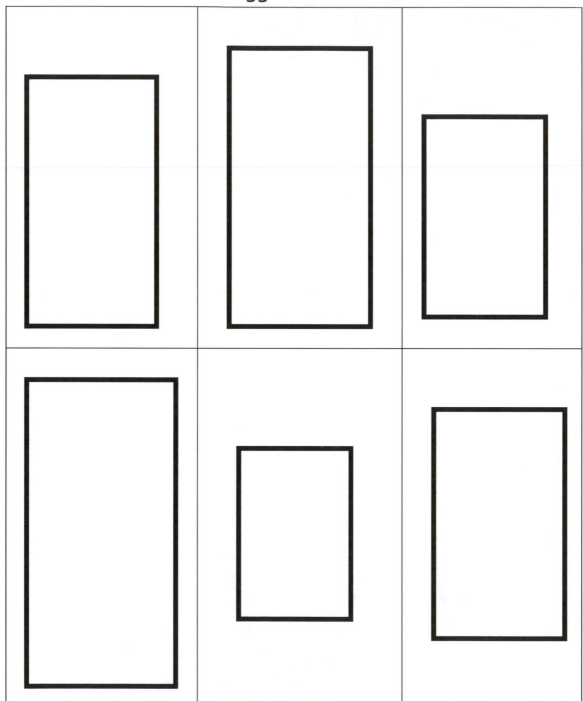

Cut out the boxes and then sort the following shapes from biggest to smallest.

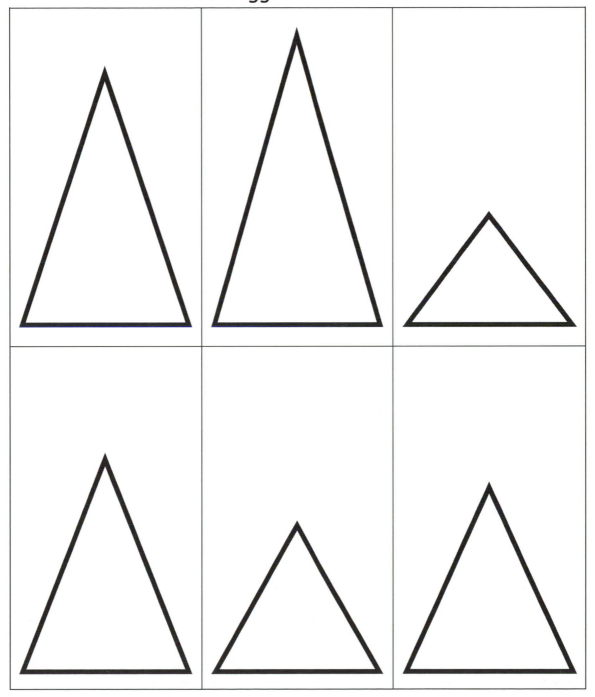

Cut out the boxes and then sort the following shapes from biggest to smallest.

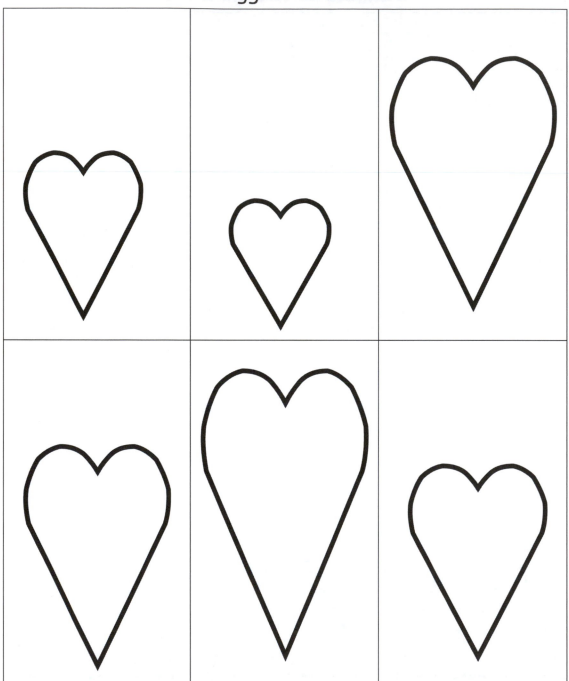

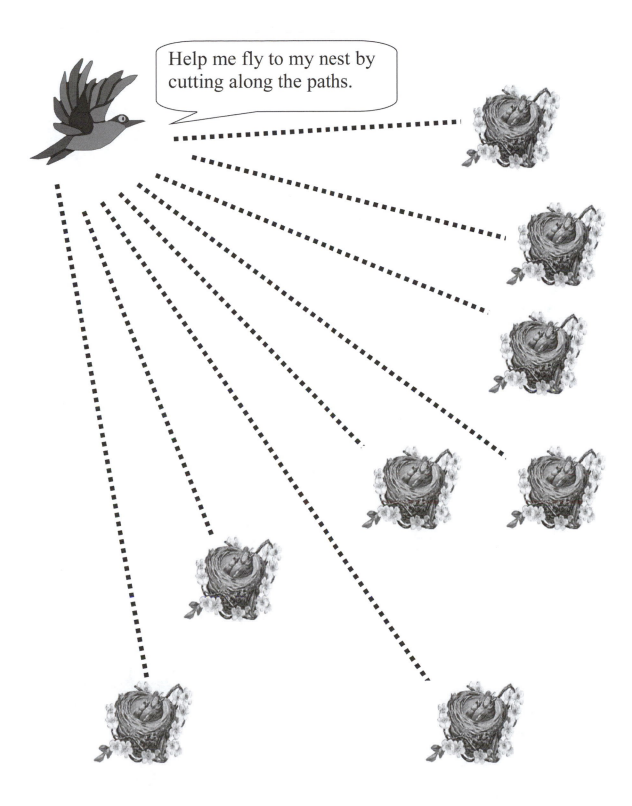

Help me fly to my nest by cutting along the paths.

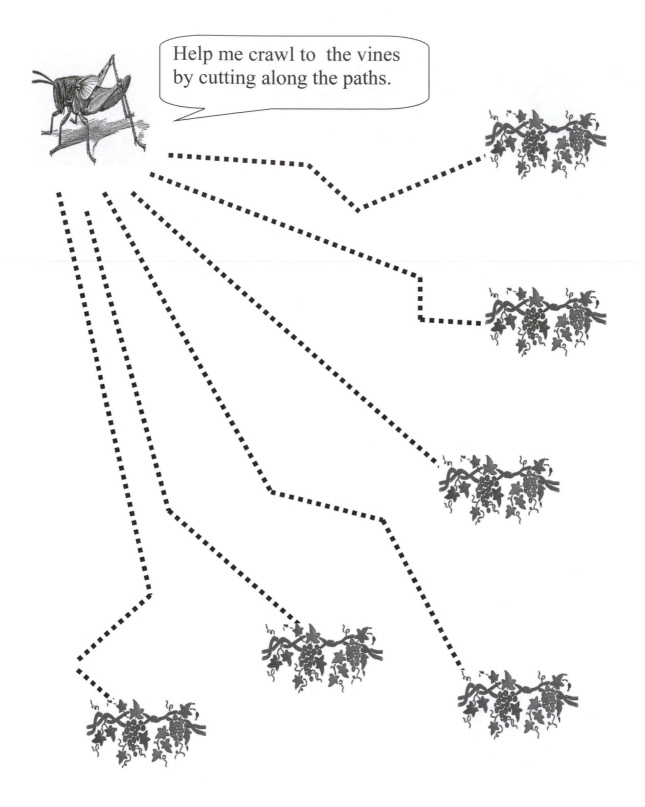

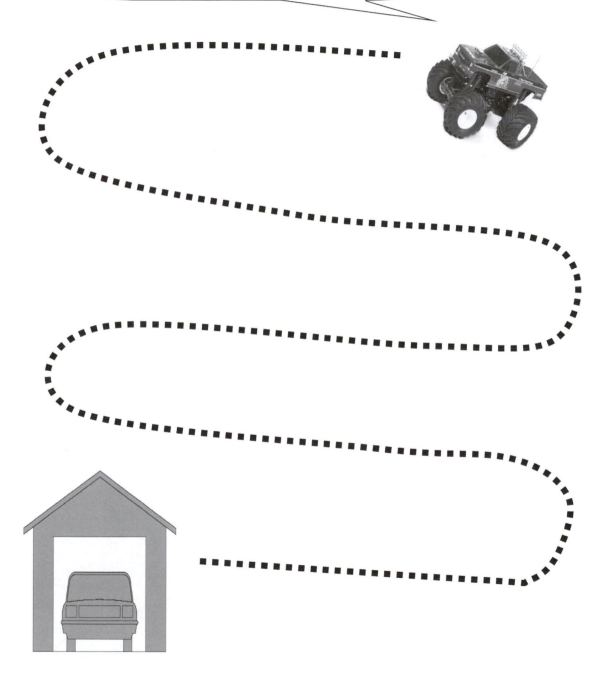

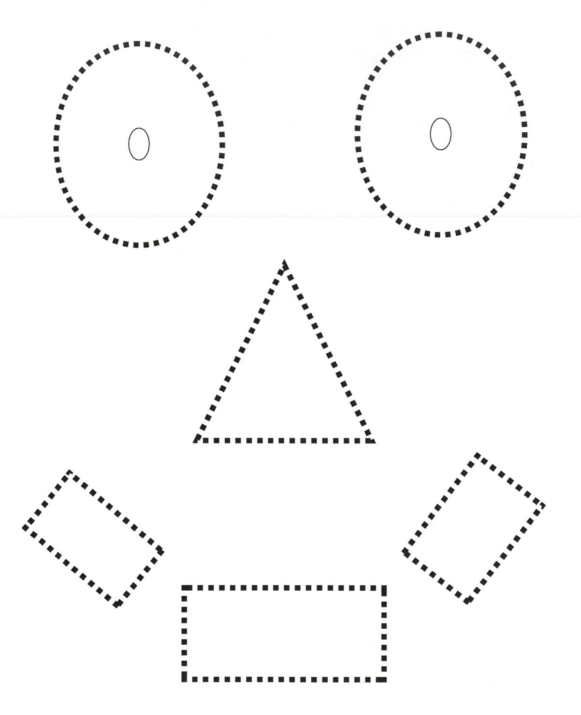

From Danto A., & Pruzansky M. *1001 Pediatric Treatment Activities: Creative Ideas for Therapy Sessions*. Thorofare, NJ: SLACK Incorporated; 2011.

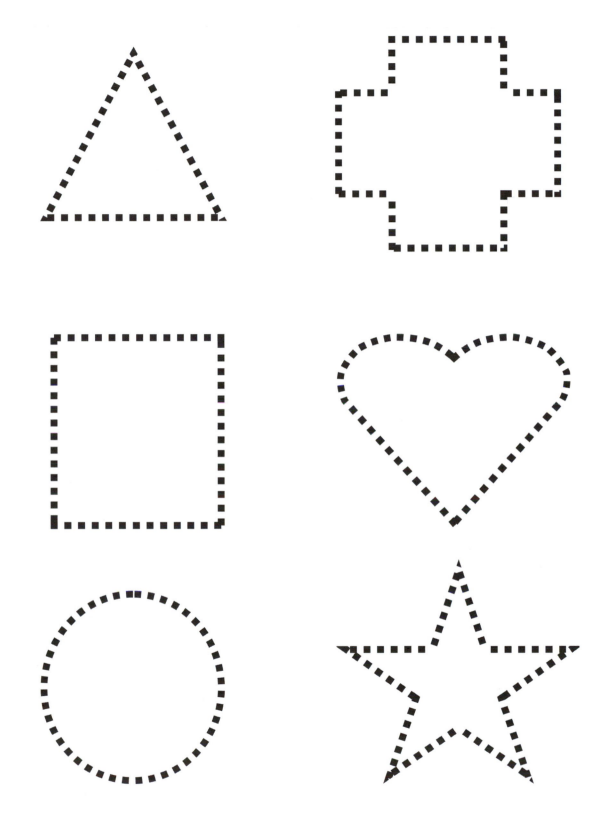

From Danto A., & Pruzansky M. *1001 Pediatric Treatment Activities: Creative Ideas for Therapy Sessions*. Thorofare, NJ: SLACK Incorporated; 2011.

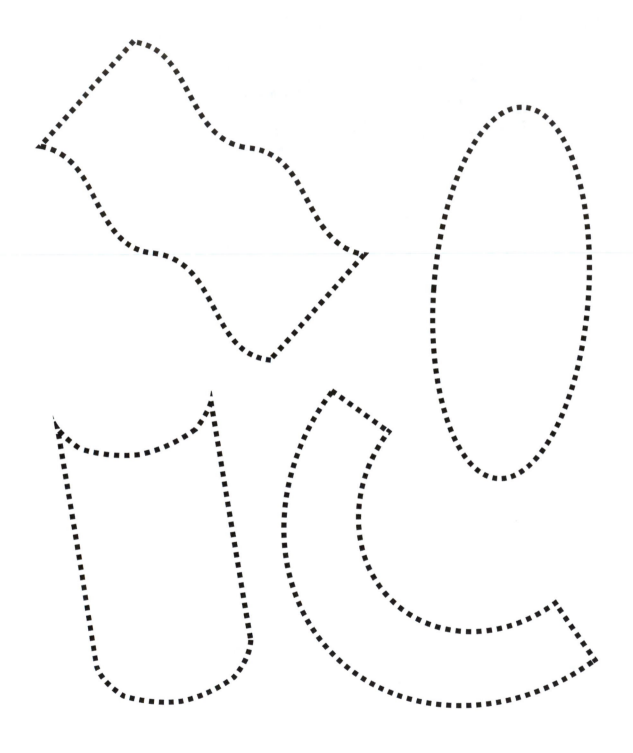

Which picture is different from the others?

1

2

3

4

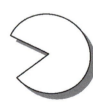 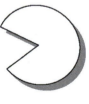 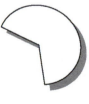 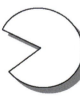

From Danto A., & Pruzansky M. *1001 Pediatric Treatment Activities: Creative Ideas for Therapy Sessions.* Thorofare, NJ: SLACK Incorporated; 2011.

Which picture is different from the others?

1

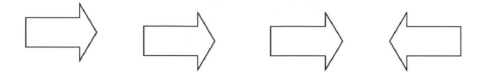

2

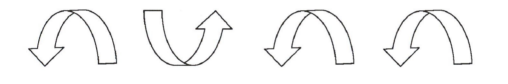

3

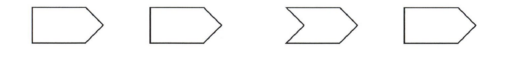

4

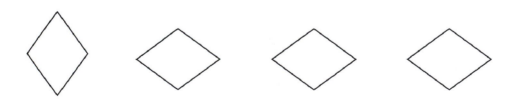

From Danto A., & Pruzansky M. *1001 Pediatric Treatment Activities: Creative Ideas for Therapy Sessions*. Thorofare, NJ: SLACK Incorporated; 2011.

Match the figure on top to the figures below.

1

2

3

From Danto A., & Pruzansky M. *1001 Pediatric Treatment Activities: Creative Ideas for Therapy Sessions.* Thorofare, NJ: SLACK Incorporated; 2011.

Match the figure on top to the figures below.

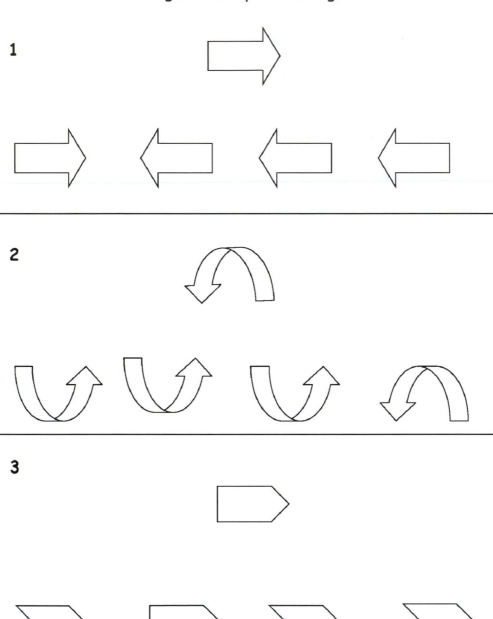

Match the figure on top to the figures below.

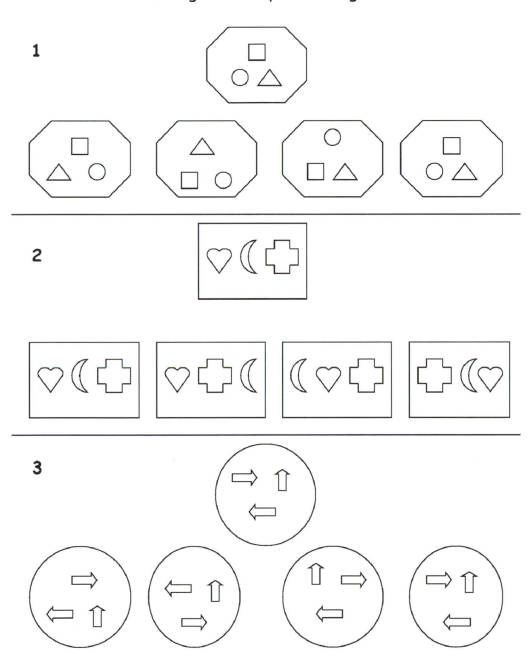

From Danto A., & Pruzansky M. *1001 Pediatric Treatment Activities: Creative Ideas for Therapy Sessions.* Thorofare, NJ: SLACK Incorporated; 2011.

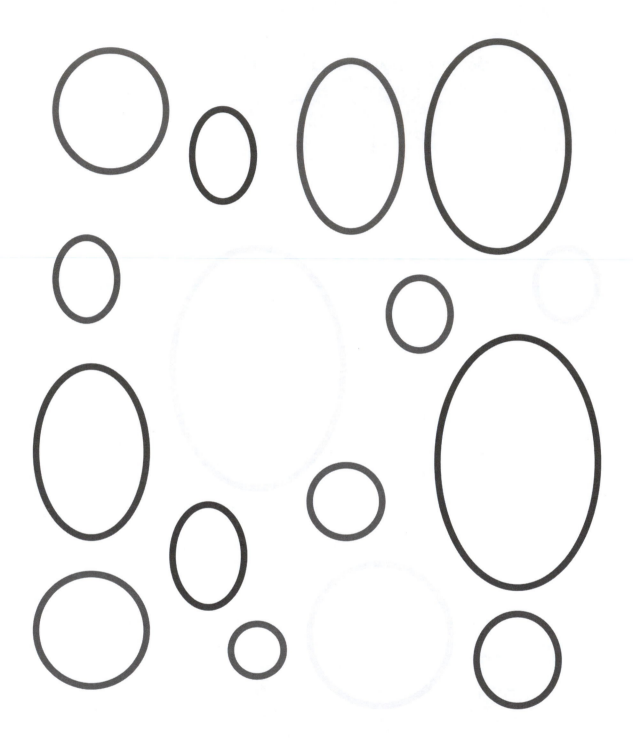

*Trace over circles with colored markers or crayons and then
use dot markers to make dots in corresponding circles.

From Danto A., & Pruzansky M. *1001 Pediatric Treatment Activities: Creative Ideas for Therapy Sessions*. Thorofare, NJ: SLACK Incorporated; 2011.

Circle all of the letter "S"s in the picture below:

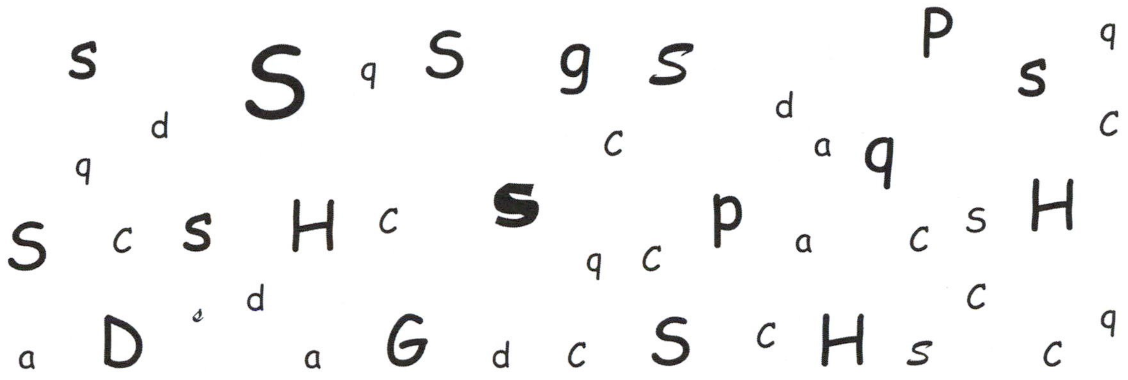

s   S   q   S   g   S   P   q
d   q   d   s
q   C   a   q   C
S   c   s   H   c   S   p   a   c   s   H
q   C
a   D   d   d   a   G   d   c   S   c   H   s   c   q

Circle all of the letter "C"s in the picture below:

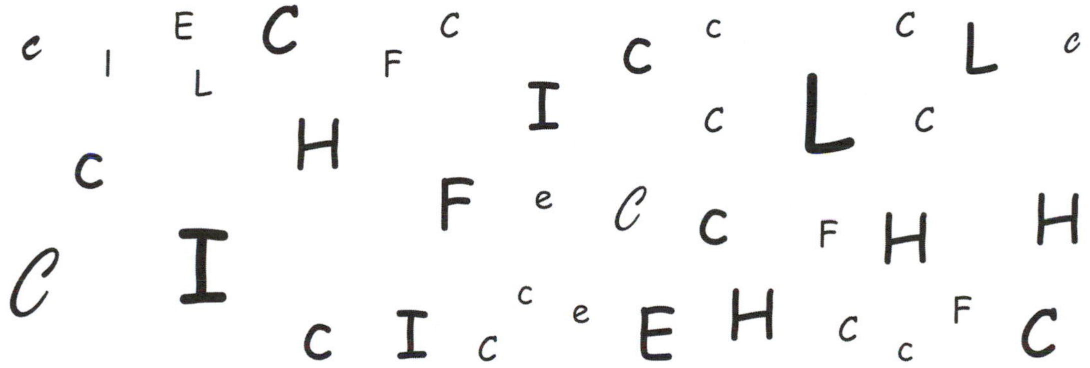

e   E   C   c   c   C   L   e
c   l   L   F   I   c   c   L   c
c   H   C   C   F   H   H
C   I   F   e   c   c   F   C
c   I   c   c   e   E   H   c   c   C

Circle all of the letter "P"s in the picture below:

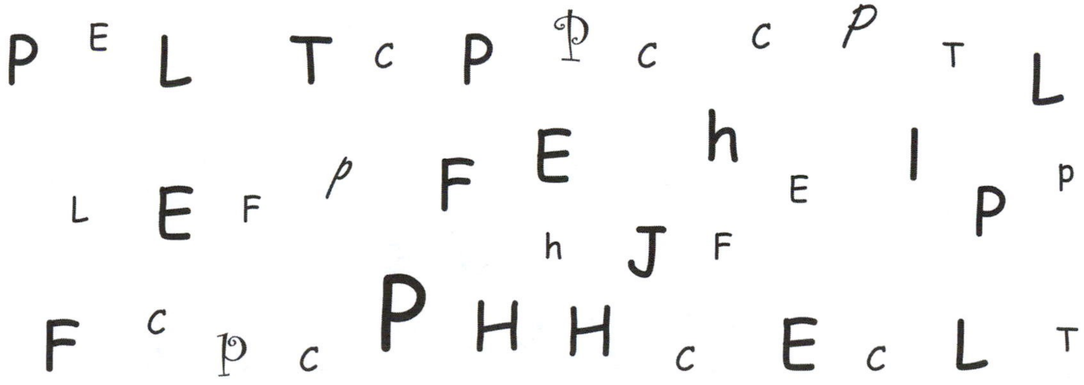

P   E   L   T   c   P   P   c   c   P   T   L
L   E   F   p   F   E   h   E   I   P   p
h   J   F
F   c   p   c   P   H   H   c   E   c   L   T

Circle all of the letter "J"s in the picture below:

j l E J F J I j j c L j

J H I J c L c

J I F e J j F H H

J I J I c j e E H c j F J

Circle all of the letter "A"s in the picture below:

a A q A G A P q

d q A P a c

A c a H c A p a c A H

a D A d a G d c A c H a c q

Circle all of the letter "Y"s in the picture below:

Y E L T c y y c c y T L

L E F y F E Y E I y y

y J F

F c y c Y Y Y c E c L T

From Danto A., & Pruzansky M. *1001 Pediatric Treatment Activities: Creative Ideas for Therapy Sessions*. Thorofare, NJ: SLACK Incorporated; 2011.

Find the letter on the top in the figures below.

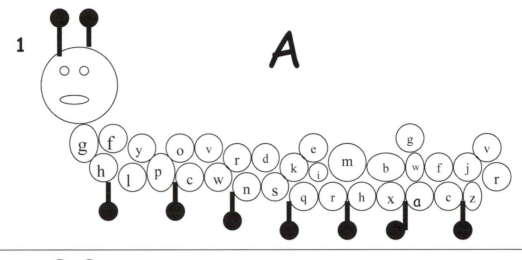

1 A

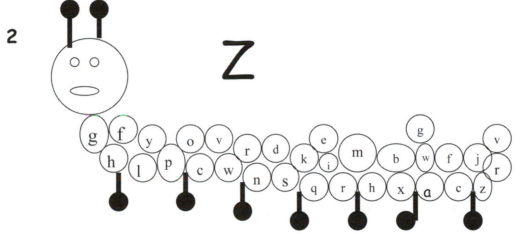

2 Z

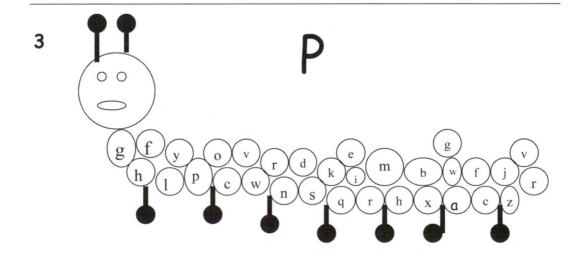

3 P

How many times does the number 17 appear in the picture below:

17   7   1   7   17   7   17   7   7

    2   2   17   12   71   9
2   9

7   3   71   6   9   **17**   71   4   1   15   17
                        0   2

82   17   4   5   7   G   0   7   8   17   4   17   8   17
                                                        9

How many times does the number 5 appear in the picture below:

5   2   8   5   5   5   5   2   7   5
        4   65

                9   25   22   **18**   11
5

        10   7   5   6   7   22   54
5   7   5   5   1   1   3   2   5   2   5
    58   6

How many times does the number 34 appear in the picture below:

34   3   34   1   2   43   3   4   34   9   34

8   43   9   5   43   3   2
    4   3   4   34   8   8   6   4

34   9   5   0   3   14   2   34   4   0   14   11

Can you guess the hidden letter?

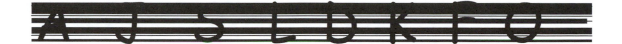

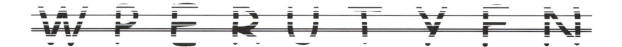

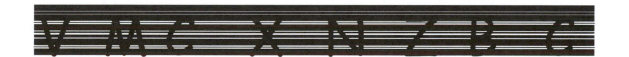

Can you guess the hidden words?

CAT   BOOK   MAP   HOT

RED   TOP   DIP   PIN

Match the complete picture on top with the choices below:

1.

   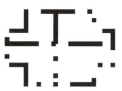

2.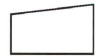

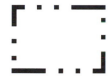 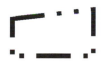

3.

  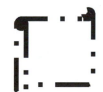

From Danto A., & Pruzansky M. *1001 Pediatric Treatment Activities: Creative Ideas for Therapy Sessions*. Thorofare, NJ: SLACK Incorporated; 2011.

Match the complete picture on top with the choices below:

1.

2.

3.

From Danto A., & Pruzansky M. *1001 Pediatric Treatment Activities: Creative Ideas for Therapy Sessions*. Thorofare, NJ: SLACK Incorporated; 2011.

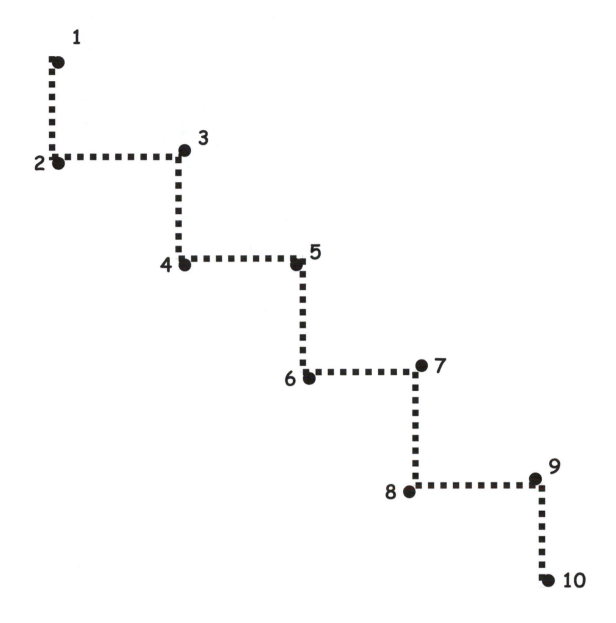

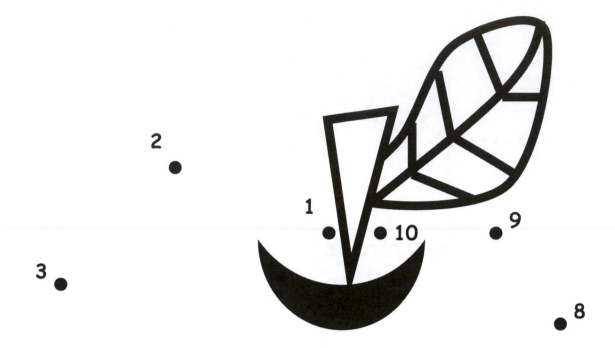

2

1

10

9

3

8

4

7

5

6

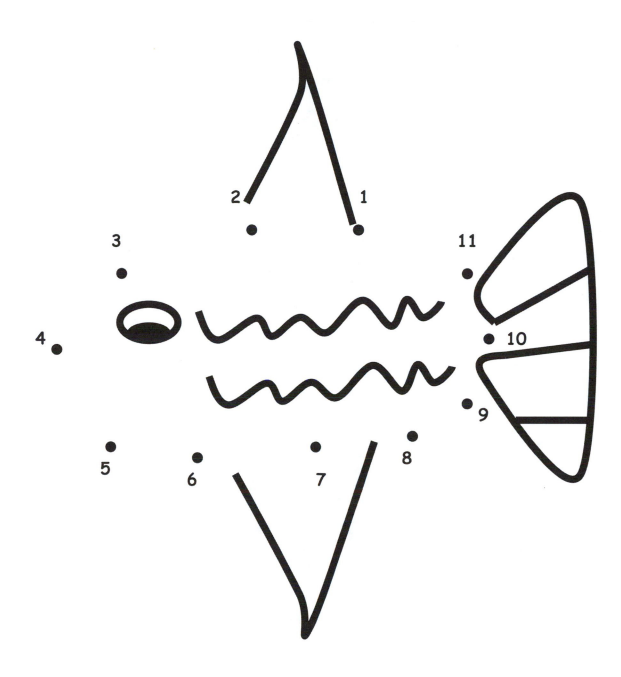

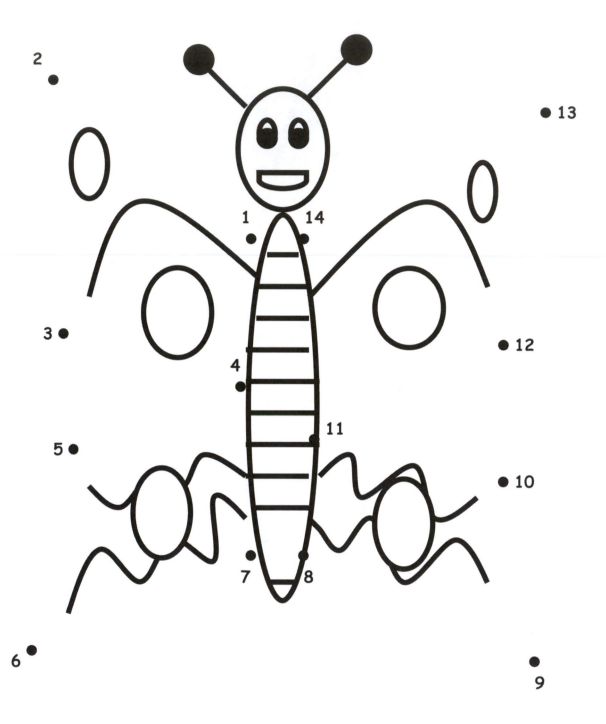

● 9

● 10   ● 8

11
●   ● 12   ● 6   ● 7

13 ●

● 14   ● 4   ● 5

15 ●   ● 16   ● 2   ● 3

● 17   ● 1

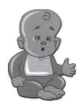

Help the baby find the bottle

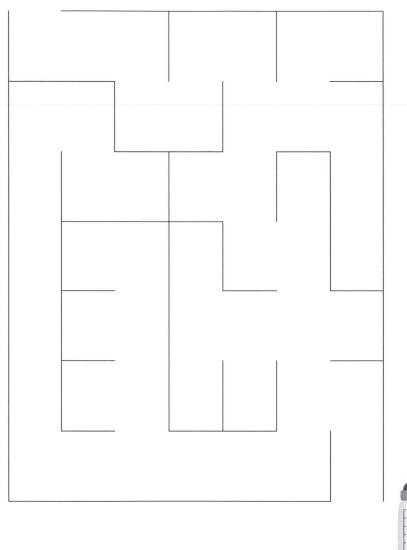

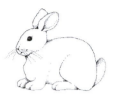

Help the bunny find the carrot

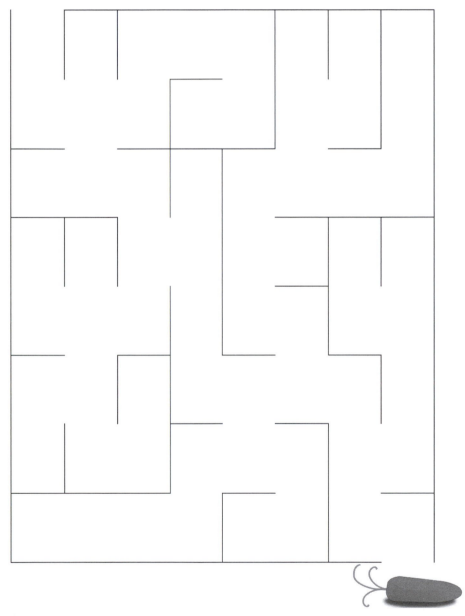

From Danto A., & Pruzansky M. *1001 Pediatric Treatment Activities: Creative Ideas for Therapy Sessions.* Thorofare, NJ: SLACK Incorporated; 2011.

Help the dog find his food

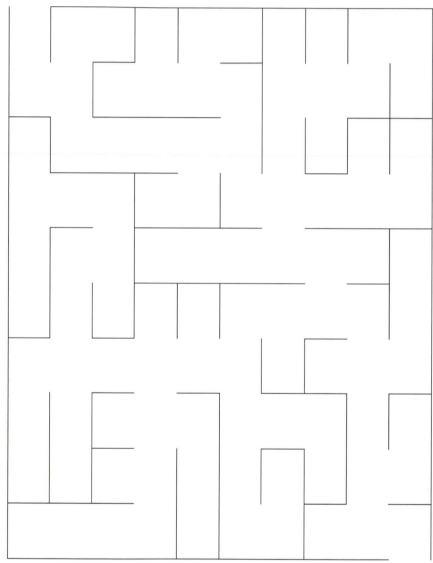

Help the bird find her nest

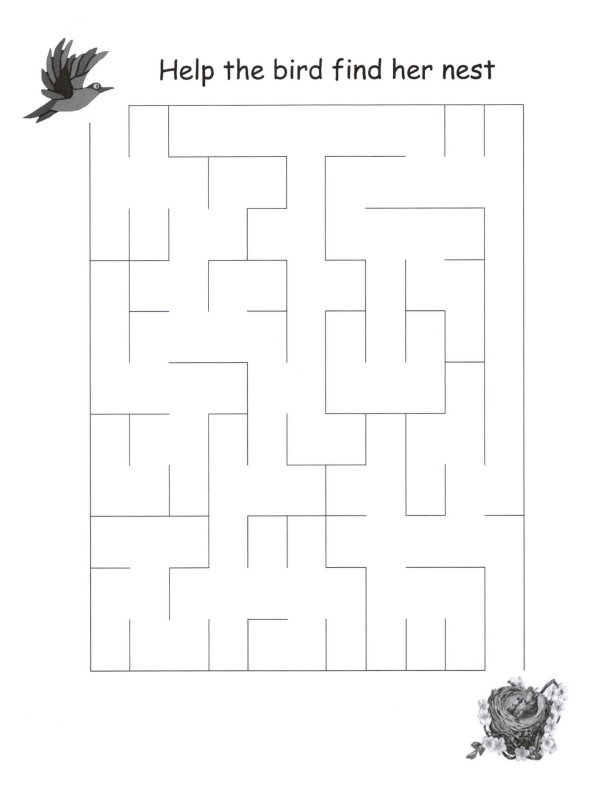

From Danto A., & Pruzansky M. *1001 Pediatric Treatment Activities: Creative Ideas for Therapy Sessions.* Thorofare, NJ: SLACK Incorporated; 2011.

Help the magician find his wand

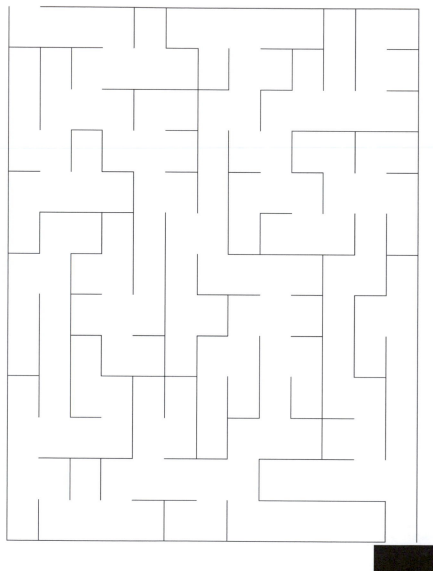

From Danto A., & Pruzansky M. *1001 Pediatric Treatment Activities: Creative Ideas for Therapy Sessions.* Thorofare, NJ: SLACK Incorporated; 2011.

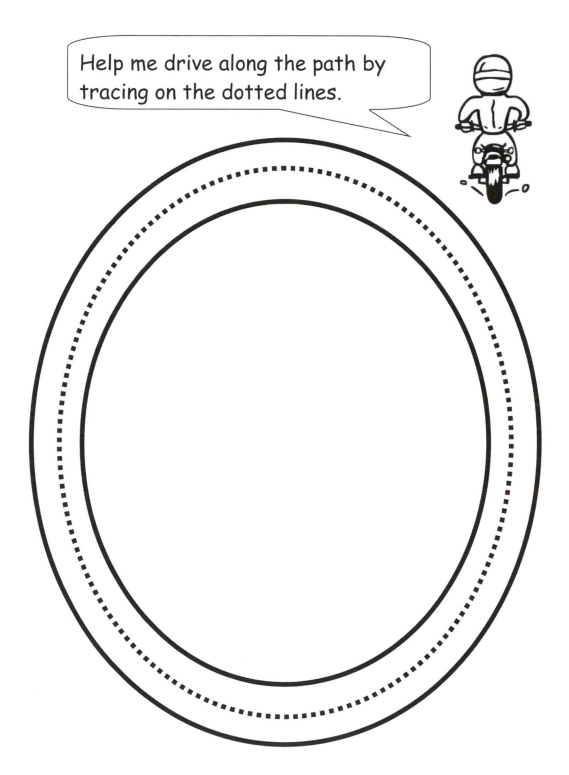

Help me drive along the path by tracing on the dotted lines.

Help the hikers get through the woods without bumping into the blocks or trees along the way.

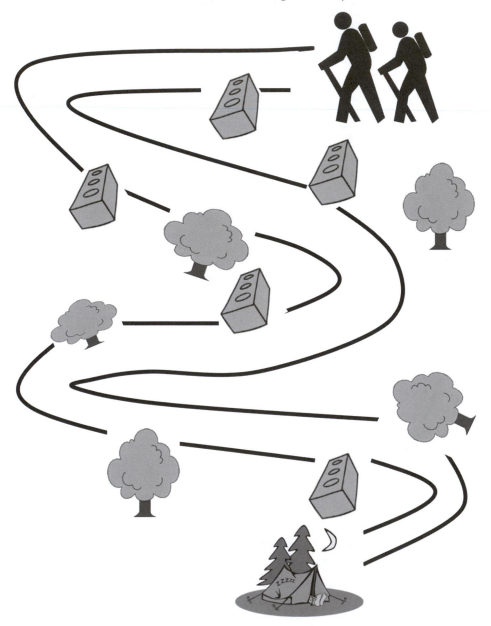

From Danto A., & Pruzansky M. *1001 Pediatric Treatment Activities: Creative Ideas for Therapy Sessions.* Thorofare, NJ: SLACK Incorporated; 2011.

Help the school bus get to school by
staying in the path.

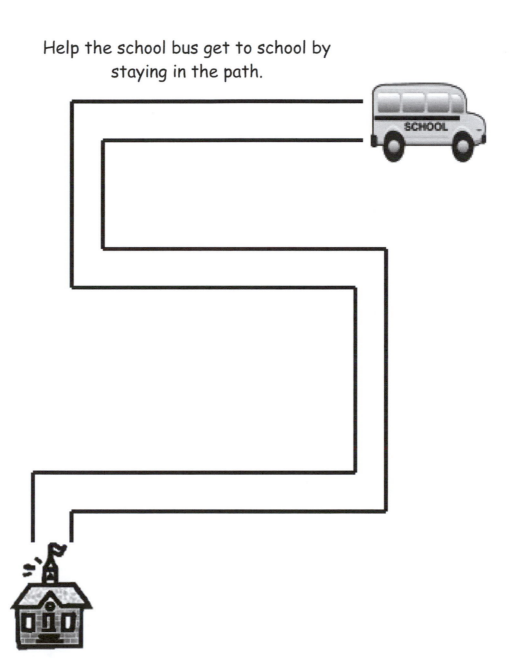

Help the girl get to the mountain
without going off the path.

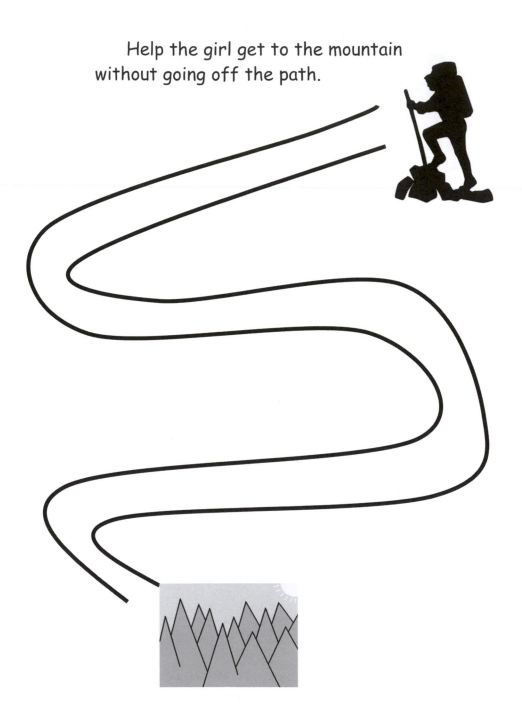

From Danto A., & Pruzansky M. *1001 Pediatric Treatment Activities: Creative Ideas for Therapy Sessions*. Thorofare, NJ: SLACK Incorporated; 2011.

Help the birthday girl find her cake by staying in the path

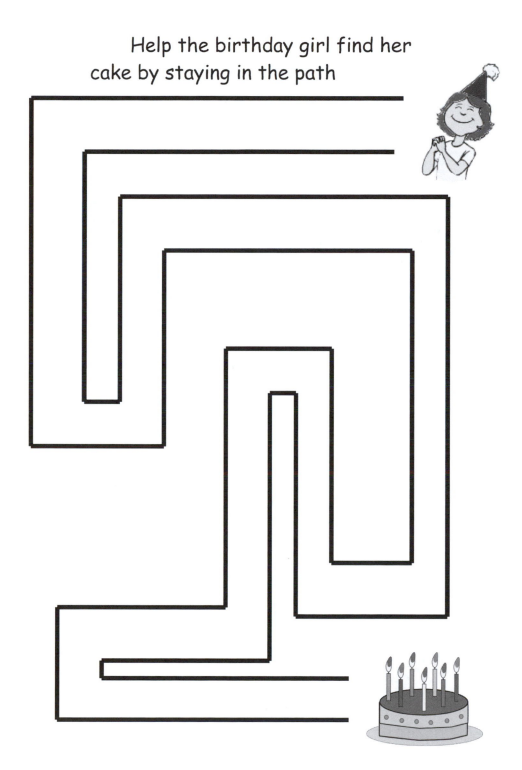

From Danto A., & Pruzansky M. *1001 Pediatric Treatment Activities: Creative Ideas for Therapy Sessions*. Thorofare, NJ: SLACK Incorporated; 2011.

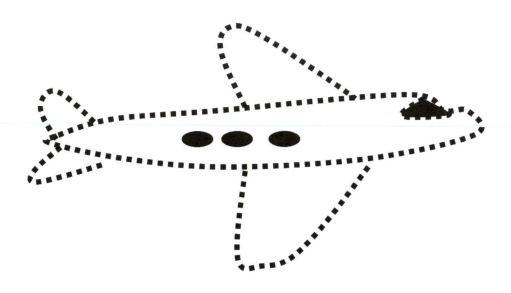

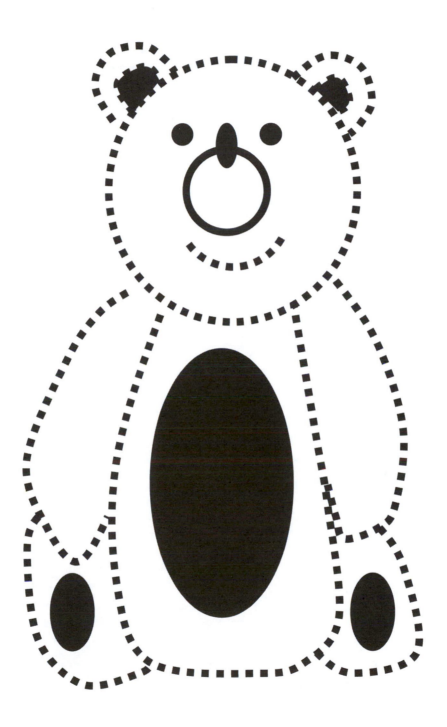

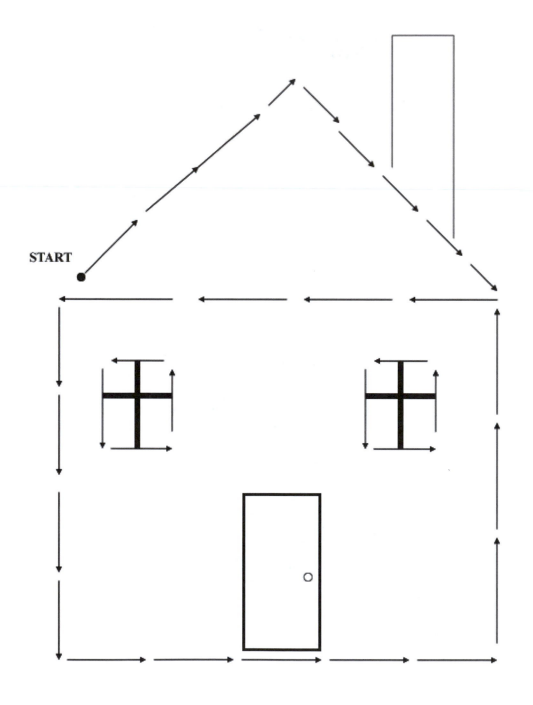

START

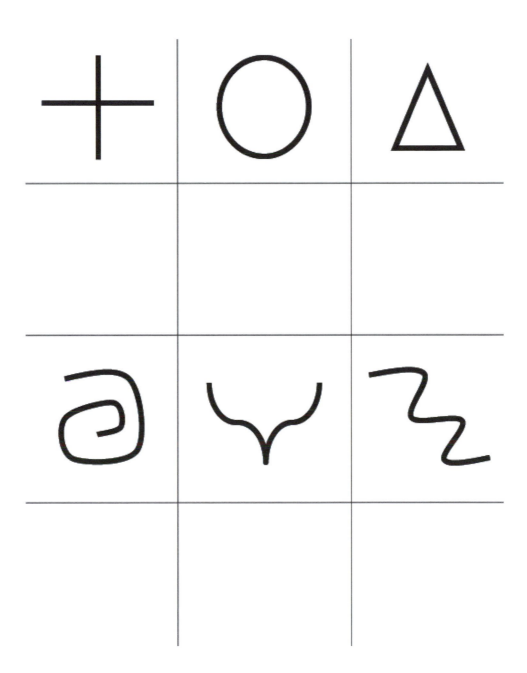

From Danto A., & Pruzansky M. *1001 Pediatric Treatment Activities: Creative Ideas for Therapy Sessions.* Thorofare, NJ: SLACK Incorporated; 2011.

H	L	G	P	I	W	Q	U	S	A
D	X	Z	C	V	B	N	M	L	K
S	W	E	R	T	N	O	P	E	J
F	C	Q	E	V	Z	X	C	H	L
I	O	P	S	D	F	G	J	P	K
U	Y	T	A	W	H	B	F	D	H
H	M	H	Z	N	D	C	Q	M	I
E	H	B	P	H	T	F	O	H	E
P	I	O	J	X	H	H	M	G	R
H	X	F	C	E	G	J	A	M	H

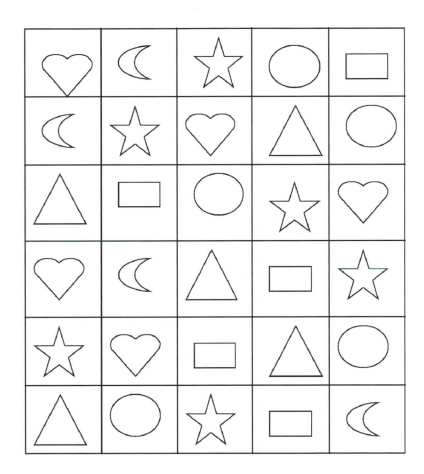

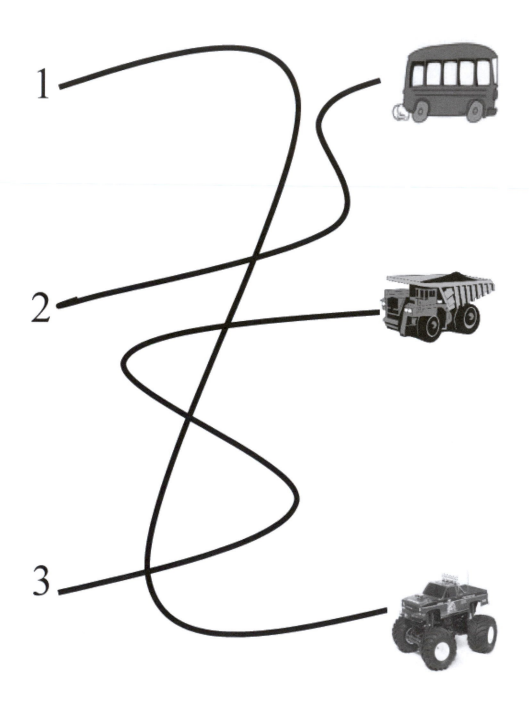

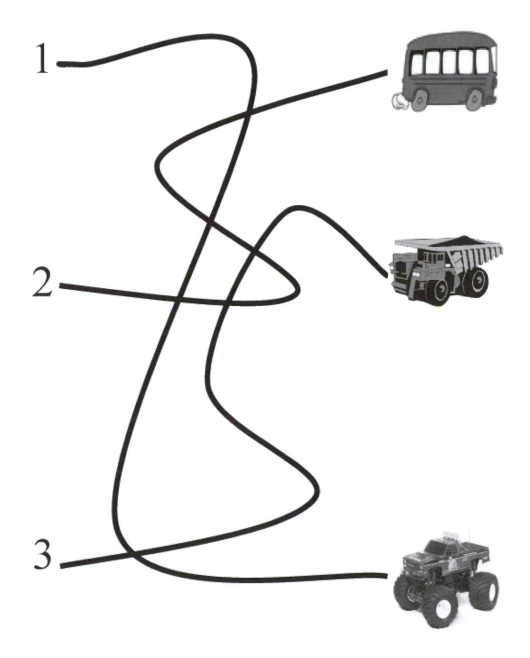

1

2

3

From Danto A., & Pruzansky M. *1001 Pediatric Treatment Activities: Creative Ideas for Therapy Sessions.* Thorofare, NJ: SLACK Incorporated; 2011.

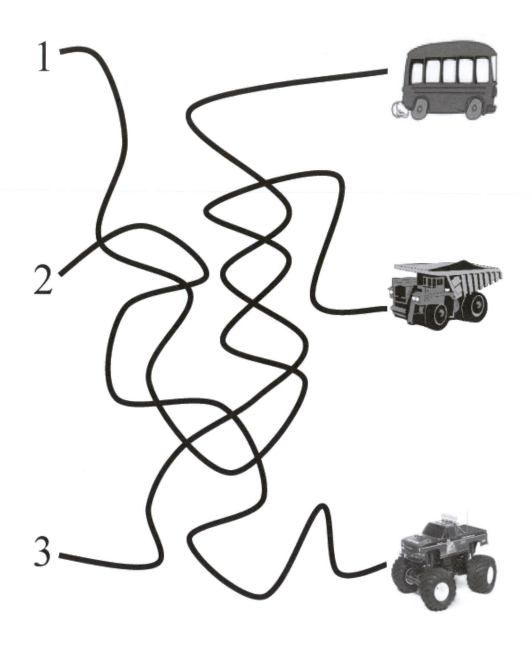

From Danto A., & Pruzansky M. *1001 Pediatric Treatment Activities: Creative Ideas for Therapy Sessions*. Thorofare, NJ: SLACK Incorporated; 2011.

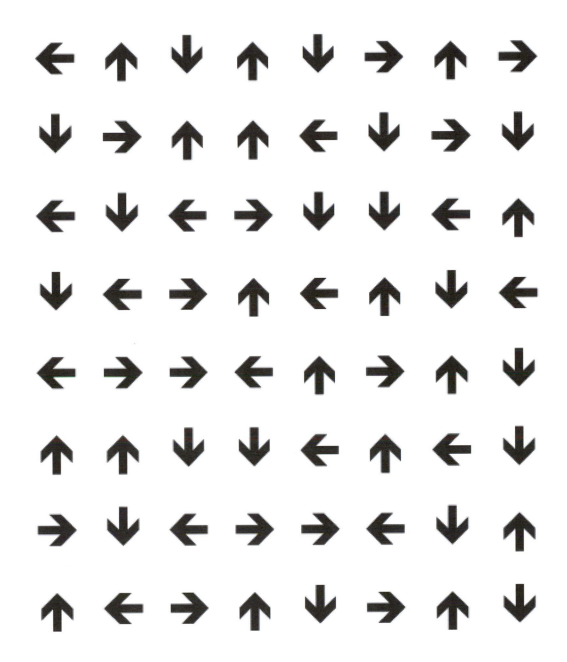

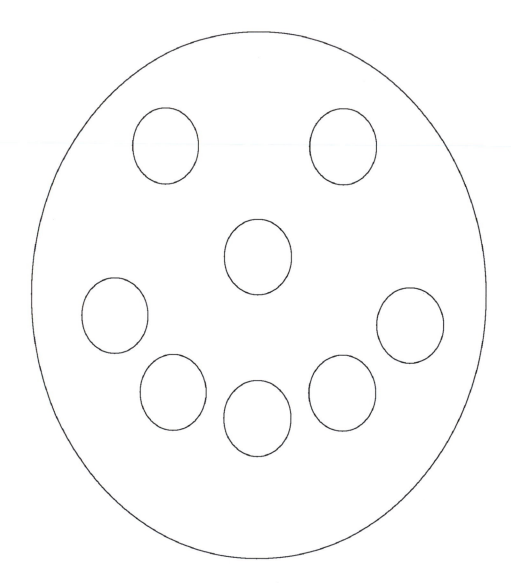

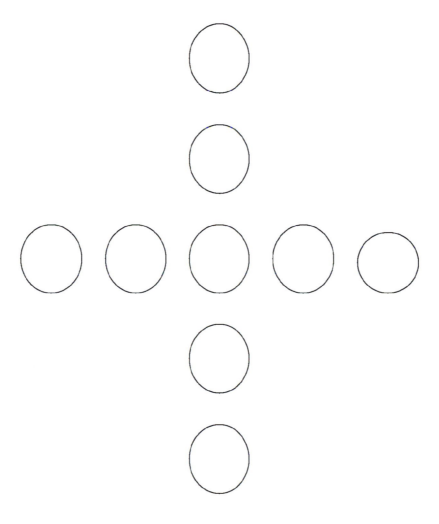

From Danto A., & Pruzansky M. *1001 Pediatric Treatment Activities: Creative Ideas for Therapy Sessions.* Thorofare, NJ: SLACK Incorporated; 2011.

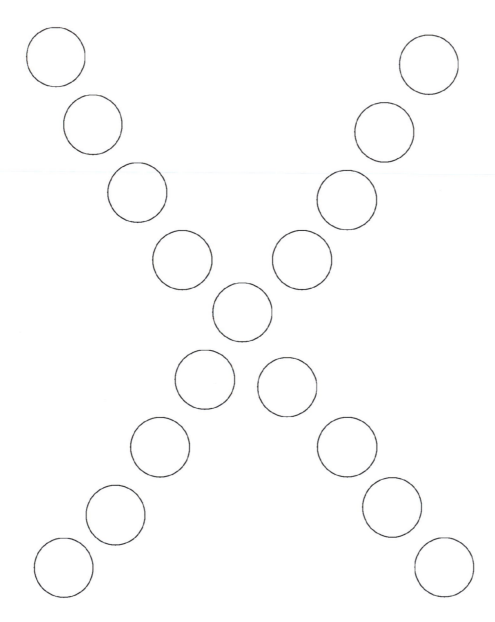

My Sticker Chart

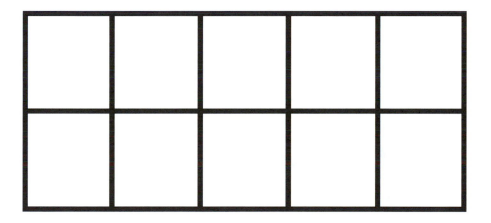

From Danto A., & Pruzansky M. *1001 Pediatric Treatment Activities: Creative Ideas for Therapy Sessions.* Thorofare, NJ: SLACK Incorporated; 2011.

Y= Yellow   B= Black   R= Red   G= Green

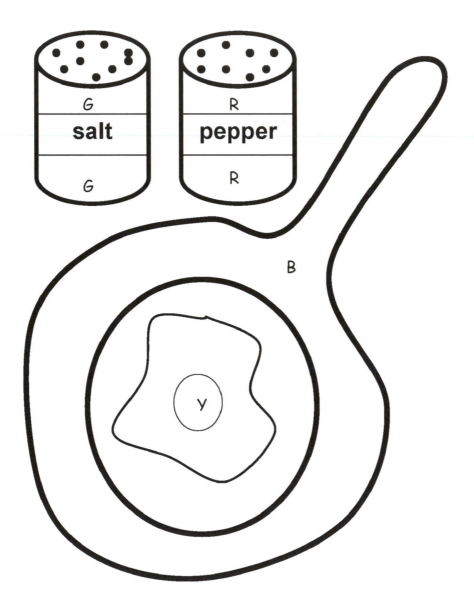

O= Orange R= Red Y= Yellow   G=Green

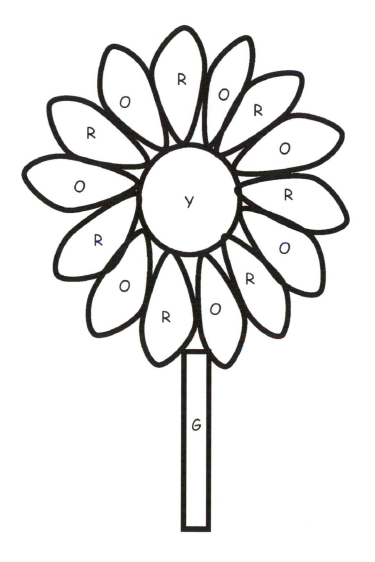

From Danto A., & Pruzansky M. *1001 Pediatric Treatment Activities: Creative Ideas for Therapy Sessions.* Thorofare, NJ: SLACK Incorporated; 2011.

O= Orange   B=Blue   G= Green   R= Red

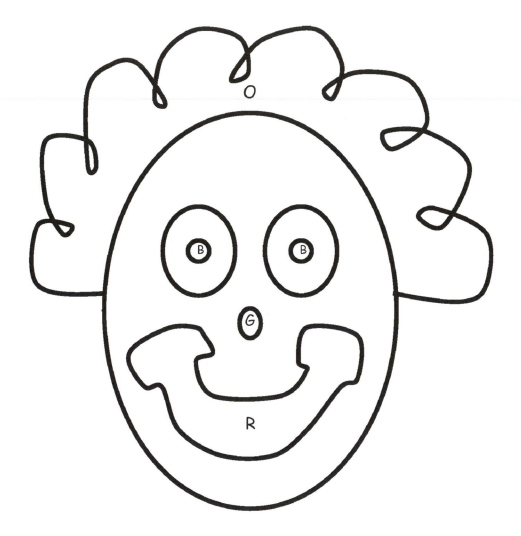

R= Red   O= Orange   Y=Yellow   G=Green   B=Brown

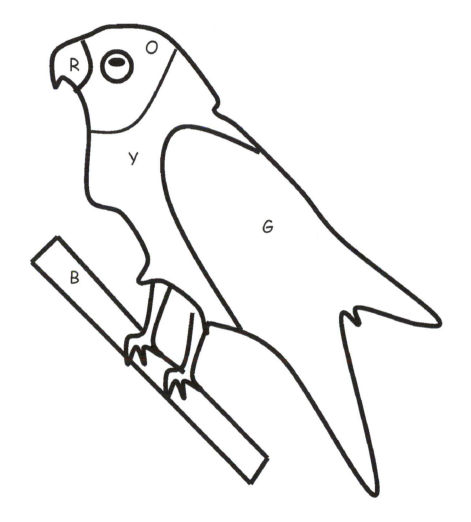

R= Red   Y=Yellow   O= Orange   B= Blue   G= Green

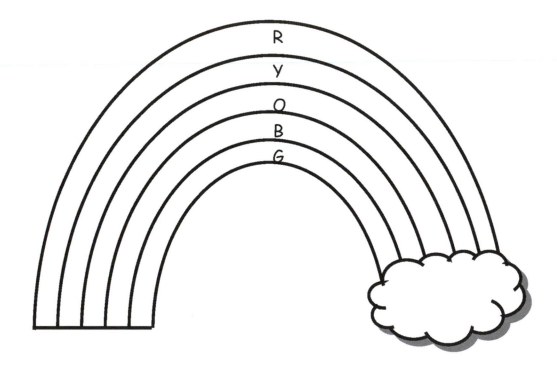

B= Brown   P=Pink   O=Orange

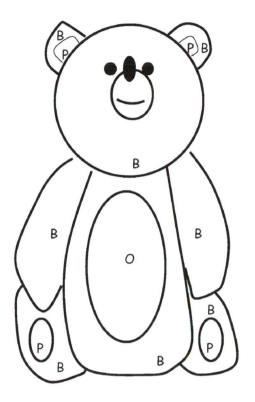

Scavenger Hunt

Can you find something ...

Bouncy
Shiny
Fuzzy
Noisy
Cold
Big
Little
Red
Yellow
Wet
Sticky
Soft
Hard
Round
Bumpy

Number Chart

1	
2	
3	
4	
5	
6	
7	
8	
9	
10	

From Danto A., & Pruzansky M. *1001 Pediatric Treatment Activities: Creative Ideas for Therapy Sessions*. Thorofare, NJ: SLACK Incorporated; 2011.

Follow the key at the bottom to fill in the shapes

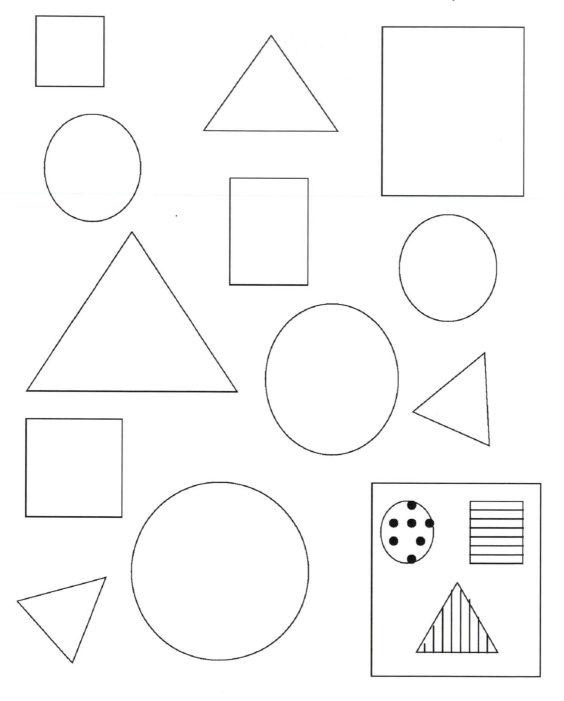

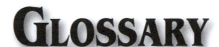

GLOSSARY

bilateral integration: The ability to use the right and left side of the body together to perform an activity.

body awareness: A person's sense of where his or her body and limbs are in relation to the environment and each other.

compensatory strategies: Strategies employed that help a person compensate for decreased strength or weak skills (e.g., wearing Velcro shoes when a child cannot tie laces).

crossing midline: The ability to reach across the body with one hand for an object on the opposite side (e.g., reaching with the right hand for an object placed on the left side).

dissociation: The ability to move different parts of the body in isolation from the rest of the body.

finger individuation: The ability to use each finger in isolation from the other fingers.

grading: The ability to make an activity more challenging (upgrade) or less challenging (downgrade) by modifying a task or demand.

input: Providing sensory feedback.

motor planning: The ability to control and navigate the body and limbs in a coordinated fashion in response to the environment and during unfamiliar and new actions.

pincer grasp: Grasping a small object between the pads of the thumb and the index finger.

pressure modulation: The ability of the body to know how hard or soft to grade pressure when interacting with objects in the environment.

prone: The position of lying on the stomach.

proprioception: The system that controls a person's awareness of where the body's limbs are in relation to the environment and each other.

quadruped: The position of being on "all fours" (on hands and knees) on the floor.

Danto, A., & Pruzansky, M. *1001 Pediatric Treatment Activities: Creative Ideas for Therapy Sessions* (pp. 275-276).
© 2011 SLACK Incorporated

sensory integration: The body's ability to take information from the environment, process it through the different senses, and produce an appropriate response.

supine: The position of lying on the back.

tactile system: The system that control's the body's sense of touch.

vestibular system: The system that controls the body's sense of movement.

Brand Name Products

The brand name products mentioned in 1001 Pediatric Treatment Activities: Creative Ideas for Therapy Sessions *are listed below, along with their manufacturer information. None of the products listed in the book or owners of the trademarks of those products have endorsed the use of their products in the manner described in this book.*

- Ants in the Pants Game (Hasbro, Inc., Pawtucket, RI)
- Ark Grabbers/Chewy Tubes (Ark Therapeutic Services, Inc., Lugoff, SC)
- Barrel of Monkeys (Hasbro, Inc., Pawtucket, RI)
- Battleship (Hasbro, Inc., Pawtucket, RI)
- Bed Bugs (Hasbro, Inc., Pawtucket, RI)
- Boppy (The Boppy Company, Golden, CO)
- Bubble Wrap (Sealed Air Corporation, Elmwood Park, NJ)
- Bug-Out-Bob (Toysmith, Sumner, WA)
- Button Candy (Necco, Revere, MA)
- Candy Land (Hasbro, Inc., Pawtucket, RI)
- Cellophane (Innovia Films Ltd, Cumbria, UK)
- Chapstick (Pfizer, Richmond, VA)
- Cheerios (General Mills, Inc., Minneapolis, MN)
- Clue Junior (Hasbro, Inc., Pawtucket, RI)
- Connect Four (Hasbro, Inc., Pawtucket, RI)
- Cootie Game (Hasbro, Inc., Pawtucket, RI)
- Cranium Hullabaloo (Hasbro, Inc., Pawtucket, RI)
- Design and Drill Activity Center (Educational Insights, Rancho Dominguez, CA)
- Dizzy Disc (Sportime, Atlanta, GA)
- Don't Break the Ice (Hasbro, Inc., Pawtucket, RI)
- Don't Spill the Beans (Hasbro, Inc., Pawtucket, RI)
- Elefun (Hasbro, Inc., Pawtucket, RI)
- Etch-a-Sketch (The Ohio Art Company, Bryan, OH)
- Fantacolor Jr. (Quercetti, Torino, Italy)
- Floam (www.discovertotalhealth.com)
- Frisbee (WHAM-O, Emeryville, CA)
- Froot Loops (Kellogg Company, Battle Creek, MI)
- Guidecraft Feel & Find Game (Winthrop, MN)
- Guess Who? (Hasbro, Inc., Pawtucket, RI)
- Handwriting Without Tears (Jan Z. Olsen, Cabin John, MD)
- Hi-Ho Cherry-O (Hasbro, Inc., Pawtucket, RI)
- Hip Helpers (Hip Helpers, Inc., Virginia Beach, VA)
- Hippity Hop (Gymnic, Lucca, Italy)
- Hula Hoop (WHAM-O, Emeryville, CA)
- Hungry Hungry Hippos (Hasbro, Inc., Pawtucket, RI)
- Hyper-Dash (Wild Planet, San Francisco, CA)
- "I Spy" Board Game (Briarpatch, Inc., Millburn, NJ)

- Image Captor (Westminster, Atlanta, GA)
- Innergizer (Newport Golf Corp, Anaheim, CA)
- Jenga (Hasbro, Inc., Pawtucket, RI)
- Katimino (Family Games America FGA Inc., Montreal, Quebec, Canada)
- Kerplunk (Mattel, Inc., El Segundo, CA)
- Kid K'nex (K'NEX Brands, L.P., Hatfield, PA)
- Koosh balls (Oddz On Products, Napa, CA)
- Lego (The Lego Group, Billund, Denmark)
- Lincoln Logs (Hasbro, Inc., Pawtucket, RI)
- Lite Brite (Hasbro, Inc., Pawtucket, RI)
- Lucky Ducks (Hasbro, Inc., Pawtucket, RI)
- M&M's (Mars, Incorporated, McLean, VA)
- Magna Doodle (The Ohio Art Company, Bryan, OH)
- Magnet Express (Anatex Enterprises, Inc., Van Nuys, CA)
- Magnetix (Mega Brands, Inc., Montreal, Quebec, Canada)
- Marshmallow Fluff (Durkee Mower Inc., Lynn, MA)
- Mastermind (Pressman Toy Corporation, Piscataway, NJ)
- Melissa & Doug Basic Skills Board (Melissa & Doug, LLC, Wilton, CT)
- Melissa & Doug Latches Puzzle (Melissa & Doug, LLC, Wilton, CT)
- Memory Game (Hasbro, Inc., Pawtucket, RI)
- Moon Sand (Spin Master, Ltd., Toronto, Ontario, Canada)
- Mr. Potato Head (Hasbro, Inc., Pawtucket, RI)
- Nuk Brush (Gerber, Fremont, MI)
- Ocean Wonders Musical Fishbowl (Fisher Price, East Aurora, NY)
- Operation (Hasbro, Inc., Pawtucket, RI)
- Oreo Matchin' Middles Game (Fisher Price, East Aurora, NY)
- Othello board game (Mattel, Inc., El Segundo, CA)
- Perler Beads (Wilton Brands Inc., Woodridge, IL)
- Peg Domino (Sammons Preston, Bolingbrook, IL)
- Penguin Pile-Up (Ravensburger USA, Newton, NH)
- Perfection (Hasbro, Inc., Pawtucket, RI)
- Picture Perfect Design Tiles (Educational Insights, Rancho Dominguez, CA)
- Popsicle (Unilever, Englewood Cliffs, NJ)
- Pustefix Bubble Bear (Pustefix, Tübingen, Germany)
- Rapper Snapper (Cleveland Tubing Inc, Cleveland, TN)
- Rock Em' Sock Em' Robots (Mattel, Inc., El Segundo, CA)
- Rush Hour Jr. (ThinkFun Inc., Alexandria, VA)
- Scrabble (Hasbro, Inc., Pawtucket, RI)
- SET (Set Enterprises, Inc., Fountain Hills, AZ)
- Silly Putty (Crayola, LLC, Easton, PA)
- Simon (Hasbro, Inc., Pawtucket, RI)
- Skip It (Hasbro, Inc., Pawtucket, RI)
- Smart Snacks Mix & Match Doughnut Game (Learning Resources, Inc.,Vernon Hills, IL)
- Smart Snacks Sorting Shapes Cupcakes (Learning Resources, Inc.,Vernon Hills, IL)
- Sudoku (Nikoli Co, Ltd, Tokyo, Japan)
- Squiggly Worms Game (Pressman Toy, Piscataway, NJ)
- Styrofoam (The Dow Chemical Company, Midland, MI)
- Super Catch (US Games, Dallas, TX)
- Tetris (Tetris Holding LLC, Bellevue, Washington)
- Theraband (The Hygenic Corporation, Akron, OH)
- Theraputty (GF Health Products, Atlanta, GA)
- Tinkertoys (Hasbro, Inc., Pawtucket, RI)
- Topple (Pressman Toy Corporation, Piscataway, NJ)
- Twister (Hasbro, Inc., Pawtucket, RI)
- Velcro (Velcro USA, Manchester, NH)
- Where's Waldo? (Martin Handford)
- Wiffle ball (The Wiffle Ball Inc., Shelton, CT)
- Wikki Stix (Omnicor, Inc., Phoenix, AZ)
- Woggler (Elrey Enterprises, Corydon, IN)
- Zoom Ball (Pressman Toy Corporation, New York, NY)
- Z-Vibe (Ark Therapeutic Services,Inc., Lugoff, SC)

INDEX

Wait...There's More!

SLACK Incorporated's Health Care Books and Journals offers a wide selection of books in the field of Occupational Therapy. We are dedicated to providing important works that educate, inform, and improve the knowledge of our customers. Don't miss out on our other informative titles that will enhance your collection.

Best Practice Occupational Therapy: In Community Service with Children and Families

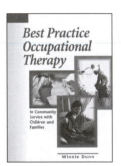

Winnie Dunn PhD, OTR, FAOTA

400 pp., Soft Cover, 2000, ISBN 13 978-1-55642-456-4, Order# 34566, **$57.95**

This book applies theoretical and evidence-based knowledge to best practice with emphasis on children and families in community settings. It emphasizes best practice, and incorporates clinical reasoning and practice models into the material.

Occupational Therapy Models for Intervention with Children and Families

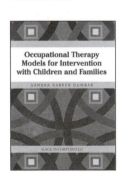

Sandra Barker Dunbar DPA, OTR/L, FAOTA

224 pp., Hard Cover, 2007, ISBN 13 978-1-55642-763-3, Order# 37638, **$58.95**

With contributions from 11 renowned leaders in occupational therapy, this comprehensive text is designed to increase awareness and understanding of theoretical models and their relationship to current occupational therapy practice with today's children and families.

Quick Reference Dictionary for Occupational Therapy, Fifth Edition

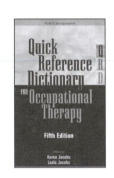

Karen Jacobs EdD, OTR/L, CPE, FAOTA; Laela Jacobs OTR

632 pp., Soft Cover, 2009, ISBN 13 978-1-55642-865-4, Order# 38654, **$39.95**

Revised and updated into a *Fifth Edition*, this pocket size resource includes the latest information in the field of occupational therapy. Inside over 3,800 terms are defined (over 250 more than last edition) and 61 appendices are included (including 7 new).

1001 Pediatric Treatment Activities: Creative Ideas for Therapy Sessions

Ayelet H. Danto MS, OTR/L; Michelle Pruzansky MS, OTR/L

304 pp., Spiral Cover, 2011, ISBN 13 978-1-55642-968-2, Order# 39682, **$48.95**

Foundations of Pediatric Practice for the Occupational Therapy Assistant

Amy Wagenfeld PhD, OTR/L; Jennifer Kaldenberg MSA, OTR/L

400 pp., Soft Cover, 2005, ISBN 13 978-1-55642-629-2, Order# 36291, **$56.95**

Please visit **www.slackbooks.com** to order any of the above titles!

24 Hours a Day...7 Days a Week!

Attention Industry Partners!

Whether you are interested in buying multiple copies of a book, chapter reprints, or looking for something new and different — we are able to accommodate your needs.

MULTIPLE COPIES

AT ATTRACTIVE DISCOUNTS STARTING FOR PURCHASES AS LOW AS 25 COPIES FOR A SINGLE TITLE, SLACK INCORPORATED WILL BE ABLE TO MEET ALL OF YOUR NEEDS.

CHAPTER REPRINTS

SLACK INCORPORATED IS ABLE TO OFFER THE CHAPTERS YOU WANT IN A FORMAT THAT WILL LEAD TO SUCCESS. BOUND WITH AN ATTRACTIVE COVER, USE THE CHAPTERS THAT ARE A FIT SPECIFICALLY FOR YOUR COMPANY. AVAILABLE FOR QUANTITIES OF 100 OR MORE.

CUSTOMIZE

SLACK INCORPORATED IS ABLE TO CREATE A SPECIALIZED CUSTOM VERSION OF ANY OF OUR PRODUCTS SPECIFICALLY FOR YOUR COMPANY.

PLEASE CONTACT THE MARKETING COMMUNICATIONS DIRECTOR FOR FURTHER DETAILS ON MULTIPLE COPY PURCHASES, CHAPTER REPRINTS, OR CUSTOM PRINTING AT 1-800-257-8290 OR 1-856-848-1000.

*PLEASE NOTE ALL CONDITIONS ARE SUBJECT TO CHANGE.

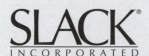

SLACK®
INCORPORATED

Health Care Books and Journals • 6900 Grove Road • Thorofare, NJ 08086

1-800-257-8290
Fax: 1-856-848-6091
E-mail: orders@slackinc.com
CODE: 328

www.slackbooks.com

1001
PEDIATRIC TREATMENT ACTIVITIES
Creative Ideas for Therapy Sessions

Keep your pediatric clients actively engaged in their therapy session with *1001 Pediatric Treatment Activities: Creative Ideas for Therapy Sessions*. Written for pediatric occupational therapy and physical therapy clinicians, graduate students, pediatric academic courses, and those in fieldwork and internships, this user-friendly guide will provide you with new ideas and activities designed to enhance your treatment session while maintaining your client's attention and interest.

1001 Pediatric Treatment Activities was written with the intent to be used among a wide range of populations and pediatric settings. Specifically, these settings include a pediatric clinic, school-based setting, hospital, and home-based therapy. This quick and simple reference is organized and written in a way that enables the user to quickly open it and skim a chapter for new treatment ideas. More than 350 photographs are included to supplement treatment activities that require further explanation. The durable spiral binding allows the book to lay flat in times when space is limited, such as in the classroom or clinic.

1001 Pediatric Treatment Activities **covers treatment areas that are typically addressed in pediatric therapy:**

- Sensory Integration
- Visual System
- Dissociation Activities
- Hand Skills
- Body Strengthening and Stabilizing
- Cognitive and Higher-Level Skill Building
- Social Skills

1001 Pediatric Treatment Activities by Ayelet Danto and Michelle Pruzansky offers therapists and students a comprehensive mix of easy-to-use therapeutic activities that they may not know exist or have not thought about including in their practice. Therapists can quickly find ideas for specific impairments and design creative and resourceful treatment sessions using the activities provided.

Each chapter includes:

- A brief description explaining the treatment topic
- An explanation of why a particular skill is important
- A list of compensatory strategies that may be employed by the therapist to assist the child who is deficient in a particular skill
- A list of treatment ideas and activities in which to engage, in order to work on the specific treatment goal
- Examples of commercial products that can be used to address the treatment goal

When working with children for extended periods of time in the same environment, it can be challenging to find and develop new and exciting treatment activities. This unique resource offers more than a thousand ideas all in one place. *1001 Pediatric Treatment Activities* will quickly prove to be invaluable to any new or experienced pediatric therapist looking for new ideas for a therapy session.

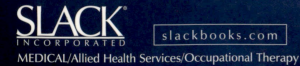

SLACK
INCORPORATED

slackbooks.com

MEDICAL/Allied Health Services/Occupational Therapy

ISBN 978-1-55642-968-2

9 781556 429682